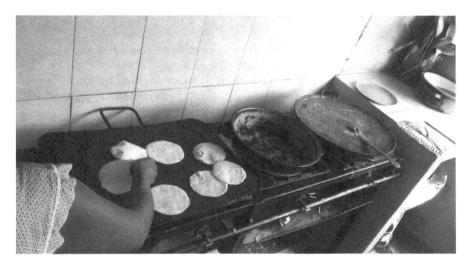

Cooking *real* food in a Mexican primary school.

From first-hand observations and deep research, José Tenorio makes it clear that school food in Mexico is about much more than feeding hungry kids; it's about how food corporations have taken advantage of social inequalities to replace native food traditions with less healthful but profitable products. School food politics, indeed!

Marion Nestle, New York University, author of *Food Politics: How the Food Industry Influences Nutrition and Health*

José Tenorio reveals how the discourse of 'healthy lifestyles' works to blame individuals for their 'unhealthy' food choices and to expand corporate market interest in the name of 'health'. This is a must-read for scholars in food and nutrition, as well as development studies, interested in understanding how larger structural forces interact with those at play at the micro-sociological and cultural levels.

Gerardo Otero, Simon Fraser University, author of *The Neoliberal Diet: Healthy Profits, Unhealthy People*

In *School Food Politics in Mexico*, José Tenorio carefully examines how the discourses of nutrition, 'healthy foods' and 'healthy lifestyles' have worked to question the healthfulness of more traditional and hand-made foods prepared by school canteen workers in otherwise cash-strapped schools, and to legitimize the interests of food manufacturing corporations.

Gyorgy Scrinis, University of Melbourne, author of *Nutritionism: The Science and Politics of Dietary Advice*

School Food Politics in Mexico

Intertwining policy analysis and ethnography, José Tenorio examines how, and why now, the promotion of healthy lifestyles has been positioned as an ideal 'solution' to obesity and how this shapes the preparation, sale and consumption of food in schools in Mexico.

This book situates obesity as a structural problem enabled by market-driven policy change, problematizing the focus on individual behavior change which underpins current obesity policy. It argues that the idea of healthy lifestyles draws attention away from the economic and political roots of obesity, shifting blame onto an 'uneducated' population. Deploying Foucault's concept of *dispositif*, Tenorio argues that healthy lifestyles functions as an ensemble of mechanisms to deploy representations of reality, spaces, institutions and subjectivities aligned with market principles, constructing individuals both as culprits for what they eat and the prime locus of policy intervention to change diets. He demonstrates how this ensemble enmeshes within the local cultural and economic conditions surrounding the provisioning of food in Mexican schools, and how it is contested in the practices around cooking.

Expanding the conversation on the politics of food in schools, obesity policy and dominant perspectives on the relation between food and health, this book is a must-read for scholars of food and nutrition, public health and education, as well as those with an interest in development studies and policy enactment and outcomes.

José Tenorio is an Associate Lecturer at the School of Human Movement and Nutrition Sciences, University of Queensland in Australia. His research and teaching interests lie at the intersection of food, health and education. He is a co-editor of the *Routledge Handbook of Critical Obesity Studies*.

Critical Studies in Health and Education

Series Editors: Katie Fitzpatrick, Deana Leahy, Jan Wright, Jessica Fields and Didier Jourdan

Critical Studies in Health and Education explores the sociological, critical and political approaches to health-related issues in education. The series underscores the discussions and debates surrounding the practice of health education and the development of solutions to the new ethical, practical, political and philosophical questions that are emerging within the field.

Social Theory, Health and Education
Deane Leahy, Katie Fitzpatrick and Jan Wright

Schools, Corporations, and the War on Childhood Obesity
How Corporate Philanthropy Shapes Public Health and Education
Darren Powell

Creative Approaches to Health Education
New Ways of Thinking, Making, Doing, Teaching and Learning
Deborah Lupton and Deana Leahy

Teachers as Health Workers
A Critical Understanding of the Health-Education Interface
Dr Louise McCuaig, Dr Eimear Enright, Professor Tony Rossi and Professor Doune Macdonald

School Food, Equity and Social Justice
Critical Reflections and Perspectives
Dorte Ruge, Irene Torres and Darren Powell

School Food Politics in Mexico
The Corporatization of Obesity and Healthy Eating Policies
José Tenorio

School Food Politics in Mexico

The Corporatization of Obesity and Healthy Eating Policies

José Tenorio

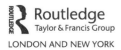

Routledge
Taylor & Francis Group

LONDON AND NEW YORK

First published 2024
by Routledge
4 Park Square, Milton Park, Abingdon, Oxon OX14 4RN

and by Routledge
605 Third Avenue, New York, NY 10158

Routledge is an imprint of the Taylor & Francis Group, an informa business

© 2024 José Tenorio

British Library Cataloguing-in-Publication Data
A catalogue record for this book is available from the British Library

ISBN: 978-1-032-41099-9 (hbk)
ISBN: 978-1-032-41100-2 (pbk)
ISBN: 978-1-003-35626-4 (ebk)

DOI: 10.4324/9781003356264

Typeset in Galliard
by Taylor & Francis Books

Para las que, pese a todo, nos alimentan;
en especial para María Fernanda, Alma y Conchita.

Contents

Figures

Preface and Acknowledgements

My mother was a primary school teacher. I grew up listening to stories about the public school she worked at in an impoverished neighborhood in Tehuacán, a small city in the state of Puebla, Mexico. One of the most common threads of these stories was food, or the politics of school food to be more precise. My mother, for example, usually expressed discontent with the management of food provisioning in the school. She also considered that food prices were high for the average student. The uses and misuses of profits from food sales by the school's leadership was also a constant matter of complaint. More than once, I heard my mother organizing her teacher colleagues to audit the revenue from the school canteen, which was watchfully controlled by a powerful, politically well-connected principal; I never knew if the audits actually occurred. What I did know was that my mother fed her students who could not afford to buy food from the school canteen. "No one can learn on an empty stomach", she emotionally said.

A national school meal program does not exist in Mexico. Multiple food products are instead sold during the 30-minute school break, which in public primary schools typically takes place at 10:00 or 10:30 am. The products on offer can range from meals made on-site from scratch to a range of industrial snacks, baked goods and sugary drinks. It is also common to have mothers selling home-made foods varying from industrial white-bread, ham and yellow cheese sandwiches to "traditional" corn-made foods. Government regulations, the local context and the economy of families shape what foods are prepared, sold and consumed in schools.

Perhaps due to my mother's influence, I became a teacher. I started teaching in 2009 in a small rural school in the state of Veracruz, Mexico. Apart from my teaching duties, I had to participate in one of the committees set up for the day-to-day workings of the school. I joined the committee overseeing the school canteen. I never imagined I was myself going to be selling soft drinks, coordinating the deliveries of products from PepsiCo and a state welfare department and collecting the quota from the women who sold home-made foods during the school break. This is where I learned about the economics of school food.

In 2010, amidst public discussions linking school food with obesity in Mexico, the principal was determined to offer 'healthier' food options in the school. Accordingly, we swapped the 500 ml-glass-bottles of Pepsi that were sold during the break for plastic-bottles of water (also delivered by PepsiCo). We also asked the group of mothers selling home-made foods during the break to change their corn-based foods—because some of them were deep-fried—for sliced fruits and vegetables. It did not go well. The students did not buy the bottled water; they brought in carbonated-sugary drinks bought outside. The price of sliced fruits and vegetables was nearly double the price of previous foods on offer. Everyone complained. The finances of the school suffered hugely. In Mexico, public schools receive limited government funding beyond teachers' salaries and, therefore, profits from the school canteen are vital for a school's day-to-day operations. The ambivalence between an idealized school food and the material reality surrounding its making, sale and consumption left me in state of bewilderment.

This book grew out of the need to know how larger forces shape what children eat in schools and our understandings of the relationship between food and health. Its writing has been a long journey. In the process, I had the pleasure to listen to, learn from and be challenged by incredible people.

I am particularly indebted to people from different organizations and institutions across Mexico City and the state of Veracruz who participated in the research informing this book. The Secretaría de Educación de Veracruz deserves a special mention. Teachers, mothers, public health officials, education authorities, school cooks, members of non-government organizations, school principals and industry representatives all contributed their share to this book. While some of them may disagree with my interpretations, I want to assure them that I have attempted to give equal value to their perspectives, even when my account is critical. I also have to say that the people to whom this book owes the most are the cooks in the two primary schools in Veracruz. I learned more from them about school food politics than from any other source.

I will always be thankful to Michael Gard for his thorough and thoughtful mentorship, and for teaching me to trust the intellectual process of writing. I am equally grateful to Gyorgy Scrinis and Gerardo Otero for helping me to refine the argument and structure of the book. I would also like to thank Doune Macdonald, Eimear Enright, Anna Hogan, Katie Fitzpatrick, Lissette Burrows and Håkan Larsson for their input on earlier versions of this book. The writing of this book was partially supported by an Australian Research Council Discovery Project (DP140102607) administered by the School of Human Movement and Nutrition Sciences at the University of Queensland in Australia.

When I was a child, I dreamed of living abroad. I wanted, among other things, to eat "other" food. As a migrant living in Australia, I developed a deep nostalgia for "Mexican" food. The Mexican community in Brisbane cured my homesickness through every shared bite. The parties, the music and the smiles kept me alive. I am equally thankful to my friends and mentors in Mexico. Despite the physical distance, they have always been there. Many ideas contained in this book were enriched by their views.

Finally, I am most thankful to my family. My mother started teaching at the age of 19. She became a teacher to overcome poverty. My father, José Manuel, only finished primary school and started working as a truck driver at the age of 15. I was mostly raised by my grandmother, Conchita, while my parents worked ceaselessly to give my siblings and I access to the opportunities they lacked. This book only exists because of their mammoth sacrifices.

María Fernanda, my courageous *compañera*, and Youssef, my spirited son, have been my source of strength and inspiration through the journey. Writing another book would be easier than finding the words to thank them for their unconditional support. *Perdonen mis ausencias. Gracias por su amor.*

Glossary

Agua fresca	In the singular, or *aguas frescas*, in the plural, are homemade drinks using different kinds of fresh fruits.
Antojitos	The way people in the state of Veracruz, Mexico refer collectively to *masa*-based foods such as *tostadas, empanadas, gorditas* and *picadas*.
Esquites	Boiled corn kernels served with mayonnaise or cream, cheese, lime and chili.
Empanadas	Deep-fried pockets of *masa* stuffed with cheese, shredded chicken or beef mince, usually topped with chopped lettuce, cheese, sour cream and a salsa.
Enchiladas	Rolled tortillas, with or without a meat or vegetable filling, covered with green or red salsa.
Gorditas	Fried *masa* pockets topped with cheese and a salsa.
Jícama	Mexican yam beam. Usually eaten in slices with lemon, salt and chili powder.
Masa	Corn dough. Used in a wide range of foods eaten extensively in Mexico. *Empanadas, quesadillas, gorditas, tostadas* and *picaditas* are examples featuring in this book.
Picadas/ picaditas	Small tortillas with a lip formed around the edge, topped with beans, green or red salsa, onion and cheese.
Quesillo	A white stretched cheese rolled into a ball. It is called either *quesillo, queso de hebra* or *queso Oaxaca* depending on which part of Mexico the speaker is in.
Quesadillas	A folded tortilla filled with *quesillo*.
Refrescos	Carbonated-sugary drinks.
Tostadas	Deep-fried tortillas topped with black beans, lettuce, cheese, cream, shredded chicken and a salsa.

List of Acronyms

ANSA	Acuerdo Nacional para la Salud Alimentaria [National Agreement for Nutritional Health]
CONADE	Comisión Nacional de Cultural Física y Deporte [National Sports and Physical Culture Commission]
CSR	Corporate Social Responsibility
CSV	Creating Shared Value
DEPE	Dirección de Educación Primaria Estatal [Directorate of Primary Education in the State of Veracruz]
ENSOD	Estrategia Nacional contra el Sobrepeso, la Obesidad y la Diabetes [National Strategy against Overweight, Obesity and Diabetes]
FUNSALUD	Fundación Mexicana para la Salud [Mexican Health Foundation]
INSP	Instituto Nacional de Salud Pública [National Institute of Public Health]
NGOs	Non-government Organizations
OECD	Organisation for Economic Co-operation and Development
PETC	Programa de Escuelas de Tiempo Completo [Full-Time Scheme School Program]
PNR	Partido Nacional Revolucionario [National Revolutionary Party]
PRD	Partido de la Revolución Democrática [Party of the Democratic Revolution]
PRI	Partido Revolucionario Institucional [Institutional Revolutionary Party]
PRM	Partido de la Revolución Mexicana [Party of the Mexican Revolution]
SEP	Secretaría de Educación Pública [Secretariat of Public Education]
SEV	Secretaría de Educación de Veracruz [Secretariat of Education in Veracruz]
SSA	Secretaría de Salud [Secretariat of Health]
UNAM	Universidad Nacional Autónoma de México [Mexican National Autonomous University]
WHO	World Health Organization

1 Governing Through Healthy Lifestyles

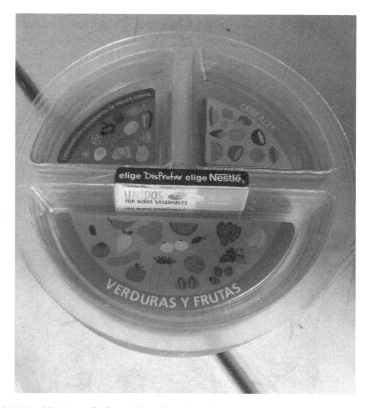

Figure 1.1 Nestlé's Eatwell Plate. Photo by the author.

On a hot Tuesday morning in April 2016, I was in the kitchen of Emiliano Zapata Primary School, in the small town of Santa Rosa, in the state of Veracruz, Mexico.[1] A couple of colorful posters featuring 'healthy' eating messages contrasted with the pale green walls of the old classroom that had been

DOI: 10.4324/9781003356264-1

converted into a kitchen in 2008. *Doña* Martha,[2] Beatriz, Moni and Angela, the four school cooks, were industriously preparing breakfast. Exactly at 10:30 am, the break bell rang. Students rushed through the front door and lined up behind the plastic table. The breakfast, Mexican-style red rice and a sour green stew, was served together on one plate for each student. This plate, known as an "Eatwell Plate", was physically divided into three serving segments: a red section illustrating meats, a green section for vegetables and a yellow section for cereals. In the center of the plate, where the three sections merged, the phrase "elige disfrutar elige Nestlé" [choose enjoyment choose Nestlé] could be seen on top of the phrase "Unidos por Niños Saludables" [United for Healthy Kids] and the logo of Nestlé, the global food corporation.

After receiving their plates and a plastic glass with freshly made *agua fresca de mango* [fresh mango water],[3] students exited the kitchen through the back door. Some seemed to be dissatisfied when they discovered that only two out of the three sections of their plate had food, and were only partially full. Others complained about the food, as they were expecting something else: any of their favorite foods made from *masa* [corn dough]. "There's one empty space", one student exclaimed. "If you paid 20 pesos, your plate would be full", a teacher replied. Everyone laughed. Although its price was very low, only 10 Mexican pesos or about 50 cents in United States (U.S.) dollars,[4] not all the students could afford to pay for the school breakfast.

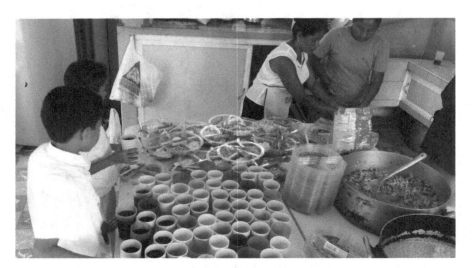

Figure 1.2 Serving breakfast in the kitchen of Emiliano Zapata Primary School. Photo by the author.

Later in the week, after a two-day fieldwork trip to Mexico City, I went to Benito Juárez Primary School, a large school located in Paso de Leones, a poor to lower-middle class suburb within the metropolitan area of Veracruz City. At around 9:00 am, I walked with Susana, the principal, towards the *cooperativa escolar* [school cooperative][5]—the name given by teachers, parents, students and administrators to the space within Mexican schools where food is produced and sold. The cooperativa escolar comprised a small room of no more than 10 square meters, which only just accommodated a Coca-Cola-branded refrigerator, a makeshift stove, two small white plastic tables and a standing potato-chip display rack. At the top of the small room where the cooperativa escolar was located, the name "Nutrilandia" was painted in big red letters; and right in front of it, another version of the "Eatwell Plate" and a "Drinkwell Jug" were painted on the wall.

Inside, a group of three women were arduously making *empanadas* (deep-fried pockets of *masa* stuffed with cheese) and *quesadillas* (a folded tortilla filled with cheese). As soon as she saw us approaching, Elena, the cooperativa escolar administrator, shouted, "We also have fruit for sale!", showing off the big, halved watermelon that she had anxiously taken out of the fridge. Her intention, as she exclaimed later, was to emphasize that she also offered "healthy options". "¡*Ay!* Elena, you don't have to pretend!", Susana said. We all laughed. Elena grabbed a piece of the *masa* used to make the *empanadas* and the *quesadillas* and said, "I also add plantain to the *masa*, so the *empanadas* and *quesadillas* are not only *masa*-based; they also contain a fruit". To convince me of the quality, taste and nutritious content of her foods, Elena offered me a product. I chose a *quesadilla*. She personally grabbed one of the recently hand-made tortillas being kept warm under a cloth, put it on the griddle, added shredded *quesillo*[6] on top and then folded the tortilla. "This is how we prepare *quesadillas*. No fat is added", Elena claimed proudly.

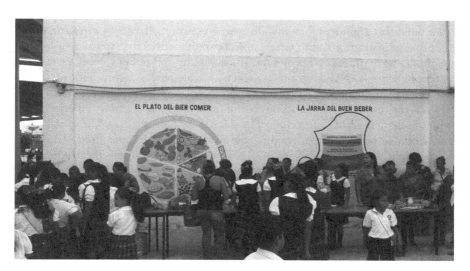

Figure 1.3 Food sale in Benito Juárez Primary School. The "Eatwell Plate" and the "Drinkwell Jug" are painted on the wall. Photo by the author.

In Mexico, the results of the 2006 National Health and Nutrition Survey (Olaiz-Fernández et al., 2006; hereafter referred to as ENSANUT 2006) positioned obesity as a vital policy problem. In response, the state, non-government organizations (NGOs) and transnational food and drink corporations launched "urgent" solutions to the problem. Underpinned by the "energy balance" premise—which suggests obesity results from an "imbalance" between "energy intake" (food) and "energy expenditure" (physical activity)—these solutions have focused on promoting 'healthy lifestyles'; that is, 'educating' people to eat healthily and to be physically active. For their capacity to bring people together and their alleged educational nature, schools have been epitomized as *the* spaces to promote 'healthy lifestyles'.[7] This book challenges this idea.

I opened this book with two fieldwork vignettes to illustrate how the idea of healthy lifestyles enmeshes within the local cultural traditions and the economic conditions surrounding schools—a point that is largely overlooked in the literature. These vignettes are also intended to situate the reader within the context under which this book has emerged: it is about Mexico, its people and their health, its politics, its education system and its manifold ways of *cooking*. Through the integration of observations and ethnographic stories from two primary schools; interviews with policymakers,[8] teachers, education authority personnel and cooks from these schools; and an analysis of policy documents and reports, this book explores how, and why now, 'healthy lifestyles' has been produced as *the* solution to obesity, and how it works in the schools day-to-day.[9] The argument I put forward is that the idea of 'healthy lifestyles' has worked to divert attention away from the political roots of obesity, and to expand market interests in the name of health by shifting the blame for the problem onto an 'uneducated' population.

To build this argument, healthy lifestyles is conceptualized as a *dispositif*, or an ensemble of institutions, discourses, objects and practices that works as a tool of government.[10] Policies and programs, the economy and politics, food, plates and posters in schools, NGOs, teachers, cooks, researchers and corporations are all part of this ensemble that has turned food into a tool to govern the health and lives of the population.[11] Although not always explicit, these "macro" and "micro" elements are connected. The Nestlé's "Eatwell Plate", for example, represents Nestlé's view that food is energy and should be measured. The plate was brought into schools through a partnership between the local education authority and Nestlé. Teachers were trained to teach the plate's message, which was, to an extent, endorsed by researchers and NGOs. The plates are material. The message they convey is discursive.

Drawing upon Michel Foucault's scholarship, scholars have conceptualized "solutions" given to problems like hunger (Escobar, 2011), poverty (Brigg, 2001; Dallorso, 2012; Ferguson, 1990) and terrorism (Aradau & Van Munster, 2007) as *dispositifs*. These analyses—mostly grounded on the integration of various data sources, as is the case in this book—have shown how the proposed solutions do not necessarily work to ameliorate the 'problem' that prompted their creation. Instead, those *dispositifs* have worked as mechanisms to deploy representations of reality, spaces, institutions and subjectivities aligned with market principles, or with dominant economic interests.

The practices of preparing, selling and consuming food in schools have become the object of government regulation in the name of 'fighting' obesity in Mexico.[12] After 2006, dozens of healthy lifestyles policies have been launched with this aim. Yet little has been said about the politics around the knowledge which underpin these policies, the forces shaping them or why they, together with the construction of obesity as a problem, appeared amidst economic policy shifts that have changed eating practices in Mexico. Building upon critical studies to body weight, food and health (Gálvez, 2018; Gard, 2010; Otero, 2018; Scrinis, 2013), this book seeks to expand the discussion, situating obesity and 'healthy lifestyles' in the political, economic and cultural realms from where they are commonly detached.

From the mid-1980s, for instance, the Mexican government started to implement a series of market-driven trade and agricultural policies that radically transformed the ways food is grown, distributed and commercialized and pre-pared and eaten.[13] In 1994, for example, Mexico, the United States and Canada signed the North American Free Trade Agreement (NAFTA). This agreement enabled food and drink corporations to enlarge their networks of production, distribution and commercialization in Mexico. With additional favorable changes in marketing and packaging regulations, these corporations started to flood Mexico with energy-dense ultra-processed products,[14] which has facilitated the emergence of obesity as a public health problem (Clark et al., 2012; Hawkes, 2002, 2006).

'Healthy lifestyles' has emerged in this context of free trade and economic deregulation. This book problematizes the emphasis put on 'healthy lifestyles' in schools as the solution to a structural problem such as obesity (Gálvez, 2018; Otero, 2018). The emergence of both the problem and its preferred solution also occurred amidst a decrease in welfare spending and an increase in private capital in previously state-owned enterprises and services, which also triggered the production of discourses through which a new relationship between the state and its citizens was channeled. As government was down-sized and market interests increased, the state's responsibility to provide care for its population started then to be transferred to individuals themselves (Howell & Ingham, 2001; Ingham, 1985; Navarro, 2007). Discourse such as choice and lifestyle, which depict individuals as rational-decision makers under ideal conditions, became more pervasive in public health and health policy.

'Healthy lifestyles' thus supposes that people can change their diets if they are told to do so, and if the environment is "regulated" to facilitate healthy choices. Mainstream public health and nutrition literature widely supports a correlation between healthy lifestyles strategies and changes in dietary habits, particularly among school-aged children.[15] Healthy eating policies, such as the ones Emiliano Zapata and Benito Juárez primary schools were subjected to after 2007, have been launched to provide students, and their families, with information on what is a healthy diet, how to choose it and its benefits. There is not anything intrinsically wrong about this message. Yet the framing of "food-as-energy" has had negative effects, and has, as this book demonstrates, aided to transfer the responsibility from a structural problem into individual hands.

One of the side effects of what I call the *dispositif of healthy lifestyles* has been the categorization of *masa*-based food as "junk food". This idea is significantly influenced by a reductionist nutritional perspective, or what Scrinis (2013, p. 2) calls "nutritionism"; an approach to food characterized by a focus on nutritional and biological dimensions of foods and by a "reductive *interpretation* of the role of nutrients in health" [original emphasis]. The problem with policies underpinned by this perspective is that they tend to exclude the social life of food. Furthermore, this reductionist understanding of food also contributes to shift the blame for obesity from its structural roots to people.

During the three months I spent in Emiliano Zapata and Benito Juárez primary schools in 2016, I observed food being prepared, sold and consumed and talked to teachers, cooks, parents and students about food and food regulations and programs. I also observed how the messages coming through those regulations and programs were adapted, adopted or resisted. Both schools, for instance, tried to restrict *masa*-based foods and incorporate 'healthier' options into their menus. This was an attempt to adhere to the directions of the *Lineamientos 2010*, a national school food policy, and to the advice of "experts" from SUMA-Nutrir, a healthy eating program developed between the Secretaría de Educación de Veracruz (SEV) and Nestlé. Trying to follow the nutritional recommendations set by this policy and program, the schools endeavored to halt the use of fats and to offer *masa*-based foods no more than three days a week. Because of the use of fats and the method of frying employed in their preparation, these foods were judged to have low nutritional quality. Students' fondness for *masa*-based foods and the local economic conditions surrounding schools, however, made these recommendations unattainable. I observed how the project of governing through 'healthy lifestyles' encountered resistance in everyday cooking and eating within schools.

According to the discourses mobilized through healthy lifestyles, Emiliano Zapata and Benito Juárez primary schools are "obesogenic environments", because most of the food options offered there do not meet the standards set by nutritional guidelines. Teachers, mothers and students can be blamed for not complying with the rules and for taking 'unhealthy' food choices, in spite of having been provided with information on how to act otherwise. However, given that my analysis also pays attention to what the *dispositif* does, this book also shows how this attempt to produce 'healthy' subjects is contested in the concrete practices of thinking and acting about food and *cooking*. When cooking, prices matter. Meals made from *masa* are ideal options to sate hungry stomachs on a tight budget. Producing *empanadas* is labor-intensive, but it only requires half the money needed for dishes like a green stew. *Masa*, cheese and fats, the main ingredients for *empanadas*, are cheap and easily accessible. Yet *empanadas* are seen as 'unhealthy'.

In making evident the side effects the *dispositif* has had on people's lives, however, I am not questioning the pertinency of the policies, programs and interventions that exist within it. In fact, this book also discusses the positive contributions healthy lifestyles strategies have had on schools. The *Lineamientos 2010*, for example, aided in the removal of carbonated-sugary drinks [*refrescos*] from schools. In Emiliano Zapata and Benito Juárez primary schools, this regulation was accompanied by the health-promotion work teachers did from the classroom while implementing SUMA-Nutrir. After 2013, children were aware of the negative effects *refrescos* had on their health. They gradually shifted from buying carbonated-sugary drinks to buying bottled water, commonly from Coca-Cola (see Chapter 6). This consumption change can be considered as a public health triumph, yet it is also a victory for corporations: they have diversified their portfolio and increased their profits through selling water in bottles.[16]

The critique of healthy lifestyles offered in this book, then, is not to discredit. It is only an invitation to think about obesity and its solutions more broadly (for a collection of works in this regard, see Gard, Powell, & Tenorio, 2022).[17] This book has also benefited from a growing body of, what I call, critical public health literature that has shown the various ways in which corporations have been shaping food and health policy globally (Baker et al., 2020; Mialon & Gomes, 2019; Moodie et al., 2021; Scrinis, 2020). It thus needs to be seen as an invitation to adopt a broader understanding of food, and its association with body weight and health in the making of policy and its research, particularly around schools.

Food in Mexican schools has multiple, often competing, roles. What is prepared, sold and consumed there is significantly shaped by taste, culture and, notably, the economy, rather than exclusively by public health goals. This is an important point. If left out of the conversation, 'healthy lifestyles' works to blame people for their unwillingness to 'eat better', and as a medium through which business-oriented views on food and health flow (Herrick, 2009; Powell, 2020). Nestlé's "Eatwell Plate" is a material representation of the discourse that constructs food as a quantifiable biological object, which is important to Nestlé. Why has Nestlé, and other corporations, had the power to strongly push this view? That answer needs some understanding of the making of neoliberal Mexico, and its relation to food, health, schools and the everyday.

Neoliberal Mexico

This book situates obesity and 'healthy lifestyles' as political, economic and cultural constructions, as much as public health ones. Their making was enabled by a series of changes in global trade and economic policy that started to be implemented in the 1980s. After three decades of steady economic growth, for instance, Mexico experienced an economic recession triggered by the fall in oil prices and the devaluation of the Mexican peso in the late 1970s/early 1980s. Pressured by the International Monetary Fund and the World Bank, the Mexican government decreased public expenditure on welfare programs, ended state price regulation, privatized public enterprises and enabled a greater flow of foreign direct investments. These measures were the conditions deemed necessary to negotiate debt and to access new loans (Otero, 1996). In a radical shift from previous economic policy, facilitated by external pressure but also by changes in the political structure within the government (Babb, 2001; Centeno & Maxfield, 1992; Gochman, 1998), post-1980s' Mexican presidents aggressively rolled out an economic and political project seeking to establish the market's primacy over Mexican society.

A well-known example is Carlos Salinas (1988–1994), who put banks, railroads, telecommunications, mining and many other state-owned companies into the hands of the private sector, and was *the* promoter of NAFTA (Pastor, 1993). In 1991 the Salinas administration reverted the land reform of the 1930s, one of the most symbolic outcomes of the Mexican Revolution (see Chapter 2). This reform removed the exclusiveness of land ownership for communities and granted corporations the right to buy, and directly exploit, the land and what is under it. Foreign direct investment increased substantially in agriculture, and other areas of the food systems. People were displaced from their communities. Rural–urban and Mexico–U.S. migration increased. Wages stagnated, and one of the main "attractions" Mexico offered to foreign investors was its cheap, good labor. NAFTA became possible due to a change in the relationship between Mexico and the United States. Before the 1980s, the form of government was framed around a nationalist perspective. In the context of the always tense Mexico–U.S. bilateral relationship, Mexican nationalism meant having "autonomy" from the United States. A semi-closed economy was, to an extent, a way of keeping the relationship with the United States manageable. Salinas was part of a new breed of politicians who started to advocate for stronger Mexico–U.S. ties, and a broader economic integration between the two countries.

Neoliberalism, as economic doctrine, was adopted to open the economy, to reduce public management in economic and government affairs and to increase the flow and profit of private capital. However, given that, as Foucault (2008) claims, neoliberalism is not merely imposing a market economy, but a broader and complex "art of government", privatizing public enterprises and deregulating the economy were just one part of the neoliberal project in Mexico. Salinas also developed a mechanism to transform politics and social organization: the National Solidarity Program (PRONASOL), a social policy aimed at alleviating poverty through provisioning food, education, healthcare and other benefits to marginalized people across the country. Beyond its apparent good intentions, scholars have claimed (Fox, 1992; Fox & Hernández, 1992; Otero, 1996), PRONASOL took 'fighting poverty' as an excuse to conduct a broader political and social transformation of the relationship between state and civil society.

With PRONASOL, the Salinas administration deployed a neoliberal governmental rationality, or in Foucault's terms a "neoliberal governmentality", that would expand beyond the economic sphere to also encompass the social sphere of Mexico's people. Olvera (2003) shows that from the early 1990s, the number of

NGOs/civil society organizations working on diverse areas (health, education, human rights, corruption, democracy and so on) grew exponentially. To an extent more social participation in political affairs advanced the democratization of Mexico, however Olvera (2003) reminds us, the idea of "civil society" has also been fundamental to push policies aiding the neoliberal project.

An illustrative example is that of the Fundación Mexicana para la Salud (FUNSALUD), a "civil society organization"—I treat it as an NGO—created in the mid-1980s between health government officials and different businesses organizations. They planned to transform the public health sector, aiming to install a pro-market model of healthcare in Mexico (Abrantes Pêgo, 2010). FUNSALUD (n.d.) is widely funded by food and drink corporations, pharmaceutical corporations and insurance companies. These funds have translated into lobbying and research to advance the interests of those donors. FUNSALUD members have also occupied top positions across the structure of the Secretaría de Salud (SSA) and officials from the SSA have worked within FUNSALUD which, as critics point out, creates clear conflict of interests.[18] Unsurprisingly, all the FUNSALUD-backed secretaries of health have pursued an agenda aligned with private-sector interests and have endorsed the research and policy proposals produced by this entity (Laurell, 2012, 2015a, 2015b; PODER, 2016).

As I discuss in Chapter 3, the increasing need for body weight surveillance and the imperative for being 'healthy' started to be delineated as shifts in public health theory, research and practice were facilitated by the adoption of neoliberalism. Mexico was not the exemption. FUNSALUD provides a quintessential example of how research has been used to advance interests aligned with this form of government. From its inception, FUNSALUD started to frame nutrition science, research and teaching in Mexico. In 1992, this organization received a large grant, which has remained active until today, from Nestlé to further develop these areas (FUNSALUD, 1994). This funded research has been used to shape health policy and to validate Nestlé's initiatives, or other times to question official policy proposals.

The set of market-driven policies we abstractly label as neoliberalism have, in one way or another, affected most countries around the world after the 1970s. Whilst it is true that many of these policies have been pre-packaged as standardized recipes in the headquarters of the World Bank and the International Monetary Fund, each country's cultural, political and social circumstances have flavored them in a very particular way. In Mexico, neoliberalism has been adopted amidst the symbiotic relationship that has been cultivated between politicians and the private sector, which can be considered as political corruption. Valdés Ugalde (1997) claims that the relationship between politics and business remained balanced in Mexico until the 1980s, when Salinas became president. At that point, political power started to become clearly subordinated to economic power, many times in favor of the interests of the political elites and transnational corporations. For instance, Morris (1999, 2009) has shown that the extended privatization of public assets personally benefited Salinas, members of his cabinet and his friends. The arrival of Vicente Fox, former director of Coca-Cola México, to the presidency in 2000, can be interpreted as the prevalence of economic power over politics. Not surprisingly, over the last two decades Mexicans have been governed by an "art of government" that is, to a great extent, dictated by and for the benefit of corporations.

My description of how neoliberalism has come to work in the Mexican context is necessarily a top-down one. My intention has been to discuss how political and economic change in the 1980s set the conditions for obesity and healthy lifestyles to emerge. Yet in this book, neoliberalism is not only an abstract, distant category, but also a discursive form that affects people's everyday lives (Ong, 2007), and therefore their food practices, in various forms.

'Unhealthy' Eating in Context

Veracruz is the fourth most populated state in Mexico. Agriculture, natural resource-based industries (oil and gas) and manufacturing are the main economic activities in the state. Veracruz is comprised by 212 municipalities, most of which are rural. The local economies of many of these places are tied to the production of sugar cane.[19]

A community of less than 2000 habitants, Santa Rosa is dependent on and structured by sugar cane farming. In 2016, during my fieldwork, less than half of the male population had permanent jobs in the industry. The rest made their living from casual jobs in the cane fields, earning roughly 100 pesos a day. Most of the women, like the four school cooks, managed their households and sought alternatives to bring in extra income. As a result of agricultural policy changes introduced in the mid-1990s under NAFTA, the sugar industry had been in sharp decline. Limited work opportunities and low salaries pushed people from Santa Rosa to cross the northern border. The parents of about one third of the students at Emiliano Zapata Primary School worked in the United States.[20] The provision of food in the school was naturally framed by these conditions. The school kitchen operated under economic pressure. The price of breakfast, 10 pesos, barely covered the cost of ingredients and labor.

Benito Juárez Primary School is located in Paso de Leones, a poor to lower-middle class suburb within the metropolitan area of Veracruz City, the largest city in the state of Veracruz. The suburb was developed in the mid-2000s, amidst corruption and environmental scandals, during the so-called Mexican "housing boom".[21] Paso de Leones was developed to cater to people migrating from rural areas in the search of a blue-collar job and to, usually badly paid, first-home buyers with professional backgrounds. As Susana, the principal, used to say, Benito Juárez Primary School is in the "rich part of Paso de Leones" because it is situated close to one of the three suburb's entrances and is surrounded by two- and three-bed-room houses inhabited by lower-middle-class families. Nonetheless, most of the students who attended the school came from the "poor part" of the suburb, where families, with an average income of under 1,200 pesos per week, inhabited tiny apartments in three- or four-story blocks situated in what looks like a concrete jungle without any leisure or green area.

Though in a different proportion than in Emiliano Zapata Primary, some parents at Benito Juárez Primary School also worked in the United States. Economic liberalization seriously affected the industrial and agricultural sectors in Veracruz. Through the 1990s, several state-owned enterprises were privatized. At the same time, the growth of per capita income drastically stagnated. With NAFTA, large parts of the rural population in Mexico crossed the northern border to become 'cheap' labor. Between 1997 and 2002, the migration from Veracruz to the United States increased by 500 percent and kept growing steadily until 2012 (Del Ángel-Pérez & Rebolledo-Martínez, 2009; Montero García & Thébout, 2018; Nava-Tablada, 2012; Pérez-Monterosas, 2012). Migrating paid off. By 2005, Mexico was receiving around US$20 billion in remittances from, the mostly 'undocumented', Mexican workers (Delgado Wise & Cypher, 2007). In 2016, remittances became the first source of foreign exchange, displacing revenue from oil and tourism (Estevez, 2016). Between 2020 and 2021, the inflow of U.S. remittances reached a historical high (Banco de México, 2022).

Not only capital flows through the Mexico–U.S. migration. Alyshia Gálvez (2018) shows how practices and understandings about food circulate in the south–north–south influx of people. Migrants adapt to what is available to eat in the United States, and when returning home, migrants bring with them the eating practices adopted in the other country. This cultural exchange has had an impact in the transformation of the diets of people in Mexico. In her 20 years of service, Georgina, a teacher at Benito Juárez Primary School, witnessed how returning migrants from the United States introduced new eating dynamics in communities and therefore schools. When she started teaching in 1996, a diet predominantly based on *masa* was still common in the small communities, and schools, where she worked. However, a range of ultra-processed products started to make their way into these, predominantly rural, schools as the 2000s progressed.

The same policies that expelled millions of rural workers from their land enabled the expansion of U.S.-based companies in Mexico, which facilitated the availability and consumption of ultra-processed products that have been detrimental for people's health. NAFTA, for example, enabled U.S. producers to export high volumes of high-fructose corn syrup, produced with subsidized genetically modified (GMO) corn, at prices lower than that of local sugar. Simultaneously, the U.S. market became the main destination of sugar produced in Mexico. While prosperous in some years, regions like Santa Rosa were subject of constant periods of scarcity caused by tariff disputes and, some would say, the industry's lack of interests to expand its supply or modernize (Aguilar-Rivera et al., 2012; Sentíes-Herrera et al., 2014). The working conditions of day laborers and mill workers—the main occupations of heads of families in Santa Rosa—have been significantly affected by the liberalization of the sugar industry (Otero & Butler Flora, 2009).

NAFTA's provisions on the sugar trade, which directly affected the working conditions of people in Santa Rosa, also motivated U.S. manufacturers of confectionery to move to Mexico to take advantage of the low costs of production offered in the country (Otero & Butler Flora, 2009). Since 2008, confectionery exports from Mexico have increased steadily, with the United States being the main market for these products (INEGI, 2021). Simultaneously, Mexico has become the second-largest U.S. confectionery export destination (USDA, 2014). Putting sugar as a commodity in the free market not only affected the living conditions of people; it has also negatively affected people's health, facilitating the conditions for increasing body weight given the high amount of ultra-processed products that are omnipresent in Mexico thanks to a greater influx of cheap and versatile corn syrup, but also to the loosening of production and packaging regulations (Clark et al., 2012; Gálvez, 2018; Hawkes, 2006; Otero, 2011).

The privatization of national industries and the increase in foreign direct investment enabled transnational food corporations to expand and concentrate power in Mexico. The sharp increase in body weight reported between 1988 and 2006 (Olaiz-Fernández et al., 2006) did not happen magically.[22] Policy changes adopted in the name of the free-market created the conditions for obesity and 'healthy lifestyles' to exist. Therefore, they are economic and political issues, as much as they are public health ones. Hence the regulation of the production, sale and consumption of food in schools needs to be theorized and researched from this perspective.

Obesity, Corporations and 'Healthy' Food in Schools

In the time I spent in Benito Juárez and Emiliano Zapata primary schools between April and July in 2016, I interacted with multiple workbooks, posters, cookbooks, cards and plates that had been introduced through multiple healthy lifestyles programs. A persistent element within them was the inclusion of the Spanish word "*saludable*". *Saludable* is one of the two translations of healthy. The other translation is "*sano*" in the masculine and "*sana*" in the feminine. Simple definitions in dictionaries mention that *sano/sana* refers to the absence of illness or a state of good health, whereas *saludable* refers to something that causes good health. Although there are some differences implicit in each word, in spoken Spanish in Mexico people commonly use both words interchangeably. As a native speaker of that language, I had never really wondered about the meanings and uses of these words, or about the politics they convey, in the context of the obesity "epidemic" as discussed in this book, until my fieldwork.

"When was the birth of the *saludable* discourse?", I wrote in my diary one day as I observed how healthy eating messages, food practices, culture and agency entangled during the break at Benito Juárez Primary School. I was sitting in a plastic chair that I had strategically situated on the side of Nutrilandia, the cooperativa escolar, and the white wall where the "Eatwell Plate" and the "Drinkwell Jug" were painted. In front of me, students were lining up to buy food; avidly eating ultra-processed products of different kinds; sharing stories and food; and others looking attentively to me. The health messages portrayed in the images on the white wall were, to say the least, being blurred as the kids ate, bite by bite, food and products that under their nutritional standards would probably fall under the 'unhealthy' category.

My fieldwork reflection on the birth of the *saludable* discourse was motivated by how the idea of *saludable* contrasted with the material practices around food in the school. This rumination was expanded by the content of the interviews I conducted with policymakers in Mexico City. During my interviews with a Nestlé's representative, members of two NGOs and a nutrition researcher, they constantly drew on the *saludable* language to argue for the pressing need of promoting "*ambientes saludables*" [healthy environments], "*comida saludable*" [healthy food] and, ultimately, "*estilos de vida saludables*" [healthy lifestyles] as ways of 'fighting' obesity. In official documents and corporate reports, *saludable* appears widely as the language guiding the direction, actions and expected outcomes of anti-obesity initiatives.

Understanding that healthy can be translated into two Spanish words and knowing how these words are used—or not used—in the context of obesity prevention is central to this book. *Saludable* was used extensively by policymakers but was barely used by people in schools. When Elena, as I narrated in my opening story, insistently claimed that the food she offered at Benito Juárez Primary School was "healthy", she used the word *sana*—"*comida sana*". The cooks and teachers at Emiliano Zapata Primary School never used *saludable* when referring to food. When, pushed by me, they associated food with health in some way, and they used the word *sano/sana*. They only used *saludable* if I uttered it first.

The primacy that *saludable* has achieved over *sano/a*, this book proposes, shows the extent to which 'healthy lifestyles' has been produced by scientists, but also by corporations. Above, I show how the *dispositif of healthy lifestyles* started to take its current form in the 1990s, as market liberalization and migration changed trade rules and diets, enabling the expansion of corporations. These corporations have become central players in the making of regulations proposing how bodies, food and health should be governed. A problematic with these regulations is their assumption that food is, above all, nutrients, calories and energy with specific biological functions, a framing that has worked both to stigmatize real, hand-made food as "junk" and has also served the agenda of corporations.

Before undertaking my doctoral training, I worked in the SEV for 5 years in different capacities. Between 2013 and 2015, as an education adviser within a school district in Southern Veracruz, I oversaw the implementation of "Ponte al 100", a healthy lifestyles program launched by the Comisión Nacional de Cultural Física y Deporte (CONADE), a branch of the Mexican government, in partnership with The Coca-Cola México Foundation. Ponte al 100 sought to address the obesity problem by "re-educating the population" about nutrition and physical activity (CONADE, 2014; Fundación Coca-Cola, n.d.). The education authorities of each state were responsible for implementing this program. School districts around Veracruz were instructed by the SEV to "impact" at least 2000 students. As proof of 'impact', we had to upload personal and fitness data collected from students to an online platform sponsored by Coca-Cola.

Although funding had been allocated and materials were produced and reported as distributed, school districts—mine included—received neither the funds nor the full set of materials required, mainly because, as Pereyra (2014) and Ochoa and Pereyra (2014) reported, the funds for Ponte al 100 were diverted both at the state and federal levels.

With limited resources, we struggled to achieve that total. By the deadline, our work had 'impacted' less than 1200 students across eight schools. Playing the system, my more experienced colleagues encouraged me to "invent numbers" and upload them to the platform to meet the required 'impact'. Accordingly, we accomplished our task in the school district. The SEV fulfilled the expectations of CONADE, Coca-Cola issued press releases to show how committed the company was to promoting healthy lifestyles and CONADE published reports about the great impact that Ponte al 100 was having across Mexico. Everyone was happy. But, beyond the 'impact' manifested through numbers, I have constantly wondered whether *we* made anything good for the health of the children? Probably not, since Mexico continues to be the top consumer of Coca-Cola per capita in the world (Gómez, 2019; Leatherman & Goodman, 2005; Nash, 2007; statista, 2013).

Of course, it would be a mistake to say that the *dispositif of healthy lifestyles* has only served the interests of corporations. Teachers, cooks and students have adapted, adopted and contested it in multiple ways. Nestlé's "Eatwell Plate" was used to serve hand-made foods that contradicted the message implied in the plate. The fact that the "Eatwell Plate" and the "Drinkwell Jug" were ignored, however, does not mean that the messages they convey were inert. During our casual chats during the school break, kids in Benito Juárez Primary School expressed ample mastery of the nutrition knowledge communicated in those materials. As they ate, or shared food with me, the students always said that fruits are healthier than ultra-processed snacks and that drinking water is better than drinking Coca-Cola. They also said that *quesadillas* were healthier than *empanadas* because they were not deep-fried. Yet, the household economy, the local culture and the wide availability, and marketing, of ultra-processed products pushed kids to prefer, first, ultra-processed products and, in second place, *masa*-based foods during the break. Bottled water by Coca-Cola was consumed at school, but *Coca*, as Mexicans refer to Coca-Cola, was always the kids' preferred option beyond this space, because they "love Coca" (see Chapter 6).

I have earlier emphasized that this book does not dismiss the public health effort to enable people have access to nutritious, local foods. I have also recognized the contributions policies like the *Lineamientos 2010* have had in schools. However, it is similarly important to say that 'healthy lifestyles' has been produced to justify that something is being done to assist the health of the population, but without addressing the broader political and economic dimensions that influence what people put in their mouths.[23] Making Mexicans return to a less ultra-processed diet, nevertheless, requires that structural changes accompany policies more focused on individual change. Through the lenses of political economy, Gálvez (2018) and Otero (2018, 2021), for example, argue that revising trade agreements and re-introducing tariffs for agricultural commodities—such as genetically modified corn and soybeans—used in the production of ultra-processed products may do more to improve the diets of Mexicans.[24]

While those changes are made, policies and programs dealing with food in schools could be improved by adopting a broader view on food. This book approaches, and proposes an understanding of, food as a social artefact (Appadurai, 1981). Food sales represent an invaluable income to fund schools' needs. Food consumption is a moment for sharing among students and teachers. Food embodies history and portrays a sense of belonging to a particular space. Beyond taste and nutritional recommendations, what children in school put in their mouths is the result of market forces and politics. Policies for regulating what can be produced, sold and consumed in schools are needed. And they could be improved if the framing of what is considered to be 'healthy' food is more contextualized to the realities under which people live.

In Emiliano Zapata Primary School, approximately 80 students, about 60 percent of the student population, ate the breakfast from the kitchen daily but only between 50 and 60 students paid for it. When 60 students paid (10 pesos) for their meal, which was the average according to the principal, the school collected 600 pesos. More than the half of that amount was required to pay for the four cooks' salaries—80 pesos for five hours of intense work. Only 260 pesos were available to buy the required ingredients to feed, at least, 80 hungry stomachs. Part of that money also needed to be saved to buy the 30kg bottle of gas that was replaced every two weeks. In the everyday in schools, discourse meets the materiality of labor and capital involved in *cooking*. Scholars studying food in schools have shown the social aspect of food provisioning and the need for thinking more broadly about how to provide students with nurturing food (Gaddis, 2020; Levine, 2008; Poppendieck, 2010). This book adds to these discussions.

Cooking the Book

What the reader has in their hands is a ready-to-be-eaten meal. To reach this final version, however, I had to read manifold recipes, source ingredients of different kinds and learn new "research-cooking methods". Policy documents, interviews and observations are the empirical ingredients of the research. The cooking of this book started with the reading of four policy documents: the Acuerdo Nacional para la Salud Alimentaria (ANSA) [National Agreement for Nutritional Health], the *Lineamientos 2010*, the Estrategia Nacional contra el Sobrepeso, la Obesidad y la Diabetes (ENSOD) [National Strategy against Overweight, Obesity and Diabetes] and the *Lineamientos 2014*. After my initial reading of the four policy documents, which is explained at length in Chapter 3, I conceived that "following" policy across the spaces where it took form, in the sense that Marcus (1995) has proposed, would enable me to unearth the forces shaping that policy. I used these documents as sources to identify potential interviewees. My initial readings took me across websites, journals, newspapers articles and other documents, where the making and implementation of policy were discussed. I identified key policy players and gained knowledge about the nature and politics of these policies in action.

I contacted these key players from Australia through emails, phone calls and LinkedIn, successfully recruiting most of them to participate in an interview.

Simultaneously, I searched how obesity policies were working across the 32 Mexican states. The state of Veracruz was one of the most notable cases doing "anti-obesity work" through a variety of forms and a plurality of organizations. I used my knowledge of the SEV and my teaching credentials, or—as people who do research within their own cultural context are named by some—my status as an "insider" (Abu-Lughod, 1991; Dwyer & Buckle, 2009) to navigate the always complicated, technical side of doing research. In this way, from a distance, I started to lay the ground to conduct some interviews with SEV officials and to gain access to schools at the beginning of my fieldwork.

A central actor in my research was Victoria, the coordinator of special programs within the Dirección de Educación Primaria Estatal (DEPE) at the SEV. From our first call in late November 2015, she connected me to other senior bureaucrats within the SEV and provided me with issues to consider in the logistics of my fieldwork. I met with Victoria in person at her office in the SEV during my second week of fieldwork in April 2016. She was a very articulate woman with extensive knowledge about schools' politics and their interactions with health promotion–related initiatives across the DEPE. Victoria suggested six schools, three urban and three rural, that I could approach. I selected Emiliano Zapata Primary School and Benito Juárez Primary School because they seemed to be Victoria's preferred "examples of success" and because Santa Rosa and Paso de Leones are conveniently located between Veracruz City, the place where I was based, and Xalapa—Veracruz's state capital, where the SEV and DEPE offices are located.

Between April and July 2016, I interviewed one researcher from a national health institute; one representative of Nestlé's Mexico; three members of two anti-obesity NGOs; six education and health authorities both at the national and state levels; three school district authorities; and six teachers, three cooks and two principals across schools in Veracruz state. I also conducted focus group interviews with all the staff at both Emiliano Zapata and Benito Juárez primary schools. Additionally, I talked informally with a few dozen parents, students, education and health authorities and workers. I opted to interview these people in line with the assumption implicit in my research question that diverse forces were driving policy.

My interviews delved into people's understanding of obesity policies, the role of schools in promoting healthy lifestyles and people's experiences in these matters. Naturally, each interviewee expressed particular ideas related to the space they inhabited. Interviewees revealed shared threads, nuances and significant contradictions around the topic. I decided to spend time observing and talking to people at Emiliano Zapata Primary School and Benito Juárez Primary School to gain a deeper understanding of how political and economic transformation, and the discourses crafted within them, affected day-to-day school food practices.

I use cooking as a metaphor to explain how I composed, interrogated and discussed the data supporting this book. I started to think of cooking as a metaphor as my data showed its centrality to my research. In my interviews with policymakers, they emphasized the need to regulate cooking and other school food practices in the name of health; education authorities described how they implemented these regulations; and teachers talked about the economy and politics of cooking. In my time in schools, as the opening stories show, I interacted with people while food was cooked, sold and eaten. I was particularly inspired by the cooks in the schools, as I observed them gracefully transforming diverse ingredients into tasty meals amidst complex politics and scarceness

Embodying Neoliberal Mexico

As a person who grew up in Mexico, and worked in education there, my "cooking" of healthy lifestyles as a *dispositif* has been rather personal; this has posed challenges and advantages both methodologically and analytically. While I observed Doña Martha cooking and directing the kitchen, I reminisced about my grandmother, Conchita. Both women were virtuous cooks. While reading my fieldnotes and attentively listening to the recordings of our conversations, the language Doña Martha used to speak about food and her devotion to cooking revived my memories of being in the kitchen with my grandmother. Like Doña Martha, Conchita never used the adjective *saludable* to describe food. They talked about flavors, colors, aromas, combinations and emotions, but never mentioned words that associated food with calories, energy or quantities.

In adopting cooking as my metaphor, I, following Denzin (1998) and Lather (1993), acknowledge that this research has been deeply influenced by my own politics, history and understanding of reality. I cannot undo the fact that I was socialized as a Mexican and worked as a teacher. Cooking, therefore, connects my history with the period where I conducted this research. I used my history to question the data. At some points, the data interrogated my history. In this story, I, as a researcher embodying Mexican culture and politics, have acted within and have been part of what I have researched. I do not intend to bore the reader with stories of my life. However, what I describe below is relevant both in theoretical and methodological terms.

I grew up within a working-class family in Tehuacán, a small city in the state of Puebla, in central Mexico.[25] I was mostly raised by Conchita while Mum and Dad worked ceaselessly to give my siblings and I access to the opportunities they lacked: their childhoods were tied to poverty and hunger. Through my upbringing in the 1990s, I experienced many of the economic and cultural changes sparked by the implementation of NAFTA and other free-market policies; the gradual dismantling of the Mexican welfare state; and the broad adoption of a neoliberal form of government. For example, the relative economic stability that my working-class family experienced for some years was greatly diminished after the mid-1990s. After the implementation of NAFTA and the devaluation of the peso in 1994, Dad started to have financial problems. The company where he worked as a truck driver was shut down. With his savings he bought an old truck and started his own business. It never went well. He could never compete against the large logistics companies that were emerging.

In the evenings, I played in the streets with my friends. My small city, like most places in Mexico in those years, was still safe. Unlike today, where the country is plunged into violence, in my childhood, kids were always outside by themselves and their parents had no fear for their safety. After playing, I used to go to the *tiendita* [corner store] to buy candies. *Don* Panchito, the owner, was a very nice old man. His tiendita consisted of an old display cabinet with some cleaning products, an old white fridge with small soft drink bottles and fresh dairy products, and an old wooden storage rack with big glass jars full of candies, biscuits and some grains and pulses such as rice, beans and lentils. Ultra-processed products from corporations were available, but I could count them on the fingers of one hand.

By the late 1990s, Don Panchito's store had been bought by a man who had just come back to Mexico after working in the United States. The man had left his hometown near Tehuacán and headed north because, like most peasants in the region, his traditional, small-scale production of corn was not profitable in the agricultural model framed by market-oriented and free-trade policies. The new owner demolished the single wooden door that Don Panchito had always opened and built a metallic fence, leaving only a small window to pass the purchases through. Petty crime had started to rise. The products available also changed. I was not able to get the "traditional" candies that I liked.[26] Instead, only cookies from Gamesa, potato chips from Sabritas and candies from Sonrics (all PepsiCo brands) were available. The store was prosperous for a couple of years. Then, OXXO stores were built everywhere; the largest convenience-store chain in Mexico, operated by FEMSA, Coca-Cola's largest bottler in Mexico. The tiendita could not compete with OXXO and was shut down.

The above stories are not only personal accounts; they have to be seen as filters through which the ideas that I put forward in this book have emerged. These stories show how the macroeconomic reforms proposed in the sake of establishing a neoliberal form of government shaped my own practices, which, even if I wanted to hide behind a "rigorous, objective" methodology,[27] has also shaped what I say in this book with regards to obesity policies, school food politics and corporations in Mexico. In writing about my place within the *dispositif of healthy lifestyles* that I have researched, I kept in mind Deleuze's (1992, p. 164) elaboration that "we belong to social [*dispositifs*] and act within them". My closeness to the *dispositif* has shaped the way I designed and conducted this research. The reading and interpretation of my data has been done from the spaces I have occupied within this *dispositif*. Aware of the implications that making a claim of this nature in the contested obesity world can have, I would say that this book has been cooked through a combination of recipes and from the inside. This process has taken place amidst a shared history between my research context and myself.

Overview of the Book

This book is an invitation to think critically about dominant understandings of obesity and its proposed solutions, the agendas behind them and their unexpected effects. Guided by the question, how, and why now, 'healthy lifestyles' has been produced as *the* solution to obesity and with what effects, through Chapters 2 to 6 I develop three sub-arguments. First, in Chapters 2 and 3, I show how the trans-formations that Mexico has experienced after the gradual adoption of economic and political policy changes aligned with the neoliberal form of government, facilitated the consolidation of obesity as a public health problem and the discursive construction of 'healthy lifestyles' as its preferred solution. Second, Chapters 4 and 6 of this book show how healthy lifestyles initiatives have been shaped by, and to an extent have aided, the interests of transnational food and drink corporations. Third, in Chapter 5, I show how the discourses that are deployed through 'healthy lifestyles' are contested in the concrete practices of thinking and acting about food and health in the day-to-day lives of schools. These sub-arguments are laid out through the next five chapters as follows.

Chapter 2 offers the reader a historical contextualization of Mexican politics and of the political uses of policy. The aim of this chapter is to broaden the current discussion that presents schools as "anti-obesity sites" and "obesogenic environments", without acknowledging the complex politics that have historically surrounded policy implementation in schools. This chapter is divided into three sections. Expanding on the discussion around political and economic change in Mexico that I started in this first chapter, the first section of Chapter 2 offers a general overview of Mexican politics through the twentieth century. This section is intended to provide the reader with information about how a shift in government and economic practices enabled the transition of Mexico from a "corporatist" to a "neoliberal" state. Drawing on this general history of Mexican politics, the second section describes how Mexican policymakers of the first half of the twentieth century used education and food policy to construct a 'modern' population and to enlarge the nascent state. This second section also shows how public health policy in Mexico has been influenced, to some extent, by the interests of the United States and, since the 1980s, predominantly underpinned by a market-driven logic. Having the previous two sections as a backdrop, the third section of this chapter explains how school food regulations changed from a "cooperative" to a "healthy lifestyles" model.

Building upon this historical background, Chapter 3 examines the language underpinning the four policies launched between 2010 and 2014 to 'fight' obesity in Mexico. Policies, this chapter suggests, are not only technical constructions to social problems; they are equally political. Policies come to exist in specific contextual conditions, and they can also be used to channel different agendas. Every word included in a policy document, for instance, is a highly symbolic device: they embody the political project of governments. Looking at how particular words are used, and the rationale underpinning them, will facilitate our understanding of how individual-behavioral-focused policies have, perhaps unintentionally, aided the expansion of corporate interests and contribute to putting the blame for obesity on the 'uneducated' population. In particular, this chapter exposes how the energy balance, shared responsibility and multifactorial discourses—and words associated to them, such as "healthy", "fight", "allies", "progress", "lifestyle", "diet", "education" and so on—have served these purposes.

Based on the premise that 'fighting' obesity is a "shared responsibility" between the public and private sectors, transnational food and drink corporations have launched myriad health-promotion programs in partnership with public departments of governments from around the world. These partnerships are often problematic due to the ambivalence between corporate interests and public health goals. There is considerable research into how public–private partnerships for health have been discursively articulated. Yet how these partnerships have been actually enacted, and with what effects, remains largely unexplored. Chapter 4 fills this gap, offering a from-the-ground perspective of how the SEV and Nestlé worked together to promote 'healthy lifestyles' through SUMA-Nutrir. Drawing on interviews with staff from the DEPE and the SEV and with a representative from Nestlé Mexico's Creating Shared Value Department, Claudia, and on observations conducted in multiple sites across Veracruz, Chapter 4 shows how this partnership has enabled Nestlé to expand its interests and to promote a narrow view around food and its relation to bodily health.

As I problematized above, the day-to-day workings of 'healthy lifestyles' in schools has been largely overlooked. Through a series of ethnographic encounters from fieldwork conducted in 2016, Chapter 5 sheds light on the unreliable meanings and significant tensions of 'healthy lifestyles' in the economically rough, and highly politicized, contexts of Benito Juárez and Emiliano Zapata Primary Schools. Analytically, schools are approached as historical and political spaces to show how internal and local community politics, funding—or the lack thereof, staffing and culture shape food practices in these spaces. Chapter 5 is divided in three sections. The first section is focused on Benito Juárez Primary School and the second one on Emiliano Zapata Primary School. Each of these sections discuss how macro- and micro-economic and political issues and culture shape the practices of cooking, selling and eating in each school. The third section argues that if school food regulations are to be more effective, they need to expand their narrow view on food and its association with health. It is suggested that more attention needs to be given to the economics and cultural significance of cooking and to the people (women) who make food exist in schools.

Drawing upon the analysis of interviews with multiple stakeholders, observations across multiple sites and policy documents and corporate reports, Chapter 6 discusses how anti-obesity policies and healthy eating programs have, to an extent, been successful in decreasing the consumption of carbonated-sugary drinks and in increasing the consumption of water *in some* schools. Yet it is also problematized how this consumption change has also served other interests beyond public health. In a country that for many years has lacked the infrastructure and the political will to provision its population with clean, safe tap water, the high consumption of bottled water can also be understood as a success for corporations rather than an exclusive public health triumph for the Mexican people.

To conclude, Chapter 7 discusses the need for alternative approaches to thinking about food and its relation to health and to the provisioning of food in Mexican schools.

Notes

1 Unless otherwise stated, the names of people, organizations and locations that were part of this research have been changed.

2 *Doña*, for women, and *Don*, for men, are titles used in Mexico to refer to heads of families or older people as a sign of respect. In this case, I used this title with *Doña* Martha because she was the senior cook in the kitchen.

3 *Agua fresca*, in the singular, or *aguas frescas*, in the plural, are homemade drinks using different kinds of fresh fruits. *Agua fresca de mango* can be literally translated as fresh mango water. Throughout the book, I use italics for words in Spanish, followed by a translation in square brackets. When a further explanation is required, I elaborate in a footnote.

4 Between April and July 2016, one USD was worth around 18 Mexican pesos (MXN). In mid-2020, the exchange rate reached 25MXN for 1USD. The rate in 2022 remained around the 20MXN. Surprisingly, the USD – MXN exchange rate returned to 18MXN at the beginning of 2023.

5 A less literal translation would be school canteen or tuck-shop; however, neither of these terms encapsulates how a cooperativa escolar actually works in the Mexican context. Chapter 2 offers a detailed description of the origins and evolution of cooperativas escolares in Mexico.

6 *Quesillo* is a white stretched cheese rolled into a ball. It is called either *quesillo, queso de hebra*, or *queso Oaxaca* depending on which part of Mexico the speaker is in. I have opted for the name *quesillo* for simplicity.

7 From 2006 to 2010, for instance, proposals to regulate food in schools and to facilitate the practice of physical activity were widely discussed in the Mexican Congress (Aguilar-Solís, 2006; Mejía-Haro & Corichi-García, 2007; Diario de los Debates, 2007, 2008). Since 2006, Coca-Cola, PepsiCo, Nestlé and Walmart have also launched myriad school-based 'healthy eating' and physical activity programs in partnership with the Secretaría de Educación Pública (SEP), the federal education authority, or the local education authorities in some states (for an example, see Plazas, 2010). In 2007, the first obesity-focused NGO in Mexico launched a "war" against obesity (Fuentes, 2007).

   In this book, I delimit education to what happens in schools. 'Education', or the need for 'educating' the population to be healthy, is widely claimed in the obesity context. Multiple policies and programs have been launched to educate people to eat better across multiple realms (for a critique of the racial politics of some of these programs in California, see Guthman, 2008).

8 Not all the people I interviewed would be defined as "policymakers" in a traditional political science sense, yet I decided to refer to researchers, NGO members, corporate representatives and government officials as such in connection to the anthropological approach to policy I drew upon to construct and think through this research (Shore & Wright, 1997).

9 I use 'healthy lifestyles', in inverted commas, to refer to a set of ideas about what is needs to be done to achieve a disease-free life. I therefore use 'healthy lifestyles' as a singular entity—a *dispositif*, theoretically speaking.

10 Foucault (1980, pp. 194–195, original emphasis) defines *dispositif* as a "thoroughly heterogeneous ensemble" of "discursive and non-discursive" elements that has "as its major function at a given moment that of responding to an *urgent need*". Deleuze (1992) further elaborates *dispositif* as an ensemble comprised of lines of visibility, enunciation, force and subjectivity. Visibility refers to the historical nature making possible the emergence of what I call the *dispositif of healthy lifestyles*, and enunciation to how particular bodies of knowledge and discourses have come to frame it. The lines of force reflect the interconnectedness between discourses, institutions and objects, and also how power dynamics cross them. Subjectivity refers to a dual process through which the lines of force subject the practices around food, but at the same time this intent of subjectification is resisted in cooking and eating in schools. *Dispositif* has been translated as "deployment", "apparatus" and "assemblage". Burchell (2006, p. xxii, original emphasis) comments that it is hard to find an English equivalent to how Foucault uses *dispositif* as "a configuration or arrangement of elements and forces, practices and discourses, power and knowledge, that is both strategic and technical". The

problem of translation has generated difficulties in applying the concept analytically and debating it academically (for examples, see Agamben, 2009; Bussolini, 2010; Deleuze, 1992; Li, 2007). With my use of the original French word, *dispositif*, I seek to avoid the static nature associated with "apparatus" and the a-historical way in which "assemblage" is used.

11 I use the term corporations to refer to food and drink corporations. I will be explicit when referring to other kind of corporations (pharmaceutical corporations, for example). Compared with other terms used to refer to these entities, such as the "food and drink industry", corporations is less politically neutral. That is why it is my preference. In the introduction to their edited volume, *Leviathans: Multinational Corporations and the New Global History*, Chandler and Mazlish (2005, p. 2) argue that the global political and economic changes of the 1970s, enabled the "multinational enterprises" that emerged "in the wake of the Industrial Revolution" to take a "mature shape" as "multinational corporations". Since the 1970s, the authors claim, corporations have grown exponentially, acquiring central roles in policymaking and even in geopolitical issues. See also Abel and Lewis (1985), for histories, empirical studies and sociological analyses of the expansion of corporations through Latin American from the nineteenth century to the 1980s.

12 I do not share the enthusiasm for using bellicose language to describe the actions launched to deal with obesity. This is why I use single inverted commas around 'fight' and 'fighting' when these words are used together with obesity. Scholars have questioned how the "war" language has been borrowed to speak about obesity. Biltekoff (2007) and Greenhalgh (2012), for instance, have argued that the "war" narrative has enabled the framing of obesity both as a personal failure and as a sign of national decline in the United States, which perpetuates a culture of fear that justifies constant surveillance over the social and individual body.

13 For NAFTA effects on food production, see De Janvry, Sadoulet, & Gordillo de Anda (1995); Foley (1995); Otero (2011); Wise (2009); Yunez-Naude & Barceinas Paredes (2002); Zahniser & Coyle (2004). For effects on distribution and commercialization, see Atkin, Faber, & González-Navarro (2018); Biles (2006); Chavez (2002); Reardon & Berdegué (2002); Schwentesius & Gómez (2002). For change in the food consumption and its negative health effects, see Clark, Hawkes, Murphy, Hansen-Kuhn, & Wallinga (2012); Gálvez (2018); Hawkes (2002, 2006); Montes de Oca-Barrera (2018); Pilcher (2004, 2013).

14 I use the term "ultra-processed products" to refer to products such as cookies, pastries, candies, salty snacks and both carbonated and non-carbonated sugary drinks that are mass-produced by corporations. The work of Carlos A. Monteiro and colleagues (Monteiro, 2009; Monteiro et al., 2010) on "ultra-processed foods" has influenced my use of "ultra-processed products", yet I use the latter given that most of my informants used the word "products" and not "food" in association with "ultra-processed". Gyorgy Scrinis' discussion of the different terminologies that have been used to refer to these types of 'foods' also shaped my approach to them (Scrinis, 2013, pp. 215–225).

15 For examples, see Bonvecchio-Arenas et al. (2010); Safdie, Jennings-Aburto, et al. (2013); Safdie, Lévesque, et al. (2013). These papers report the effectiveness of an anti-obesity intervention in "improving" the "school food environment and child healthy behaviours". The study was conducted in 12 primary schools in Mexico City. The project was funded by the Pan American Health Organization (PAHO), the Mexican government and by the International Life Sciences Institute's (ILSI) program "Healthy Lifestyles, Healthy People" co-developed between ILSI and the U.S. Centers for Disease Control and Prevention (CDC). ILSI is a corporate-funded non-profit organization that has been widely accused of shaping policy for corporate benefit (see Greenhalgh, 2021; Lougheed, 2006; Mialon et al., 2021; Nestle, 2015).

16 Tap water is not always suitable for human consumption in Mexico. Although it is difficult to know whether all running water in Mexico is contaminated, multiple studies

have shown that tap water does not usually meet the criteria to be considered safe for human consumption. For a compilation of these studies, see Mazari-Hiriart et al. (2010).

17 I approach obesity from a socio-critical perspective (see Powell et al., 2022). Drawing on the work of historians (Sant'Anna, 2016; Schwartz, 1986; Stearns, 1997), epidemiologists (Flegal, 2022; Flegal et al., 2005, 2019) and sociologists (Gard, 2010; Gard & Wright, 2005; Guthman, 2011; Patel, 2009; Saguy & Riley, 2005), I acknowledge that the construction of body weight as a disease has emerged at the intersection of heated scientific debates, moral assumptions, complex politics and economic interests. Yet by adopting this view, I am not arguing that obesity does not exist or am I questioning the evidence that supports this idea.. In fact, the analysis proposed in this book rests upon the assumption that obesity *is* a problem in Mexico. However, rather than focusing on blaming individuals for their incapacity to be 'healthy'—and therefore thin, I approach obesity as the direct result of market-driven economic and political policy (Gálvez, 2018; Guthman, 2022; Otero, 2018).

18 The power of this organisation in health policy and practice is expressed by the fact that, from the time of its creation, a FUNSALUD member has occupied the SSA director's seat. Blanes i Vidal et al. (2012) call this movement from government service into private practice a "revolving door", suggesting that the private sector benefits considerably from this phenomenon, gaining access to top information and contacts acquired through, and with resources from, the public sector.

19 The research informing the healthy lifestyles strategies discussed here was produced in settings in Mexico City by researchers working in, or close to, this place. Culturally speaking, Mexico is a bricolage, which many times is not considering in policy making. I offer a perspective from the "periphery" to enrich our understanding of how diverse social, economic and political context shape the implementation of healthy lifestyles strategies.

20 Del Ángel-Pérez and Rebolledo-Martínez (2009) and Pérez-Monterosas (2012) have shown that the sharp decline in the sugar and coffee industries in central Veracruz intensified migration to the United States from mid-1990s.

21 Reyes (2020, p. 504) argues that the housing model of providing "state-assured financial security [to] enlarge private revenues" is an example of how "market power and neoliberal excess" have prevailed over the interest of the population in Mexico. Other research has documented how private developers profited from mass-producing small, nearly identical houses lacking services and with poor infrastructure built during the "housing boom" (Ascencio Ramos, 2019; Harner, Jiménez Huerta, & Cruz Solís, 2009; Inclán Valadez, 2013).

22 In 1988, the prevalence of combined overweight and obesity in adult women was 34.5 percent, a number that grew exponentially to 61 percent in 1999. This survey also reported that the combined prevalence of obesity and overweight among school-aged children increased from 18.6 percent in 1999 to 39.7 percent in 2006.

23 By now, I could be accused of not acknowledging that school-based healthy eating policies sit within a broader, complementary anti-obesity policy framework that seeks to create "healthy environments" where people can take "informed choices". The "sugar tax" that has been in place since 2014 and the food labelling regulation that was passed in 2019 are policies aimed at modifying the environment, but they still boil down to ensuring positive decision-making by individuals, an approach that might be not the best in a country where the consumption of ultra-processed products is rooted in culture and is many times a sign of class distinction (see Jenatton & Morales, 2020).

24 Gálvez and Otero convincingly argue how structural solutions may improve the diets of Mexican people, yet they fail to empirically demonstrate how behavioral change-focused solutions work to transform systematic failure into individual failure. Chapters 4, 5 and 6 of this book fill this gap.

25 When I was a kid, my mother, a teacher, always told me to say at school that we were a "lower-middle-class family". While this class membership was probably true until the mid-1990s, this changed afterwards, when my father, a truck-driver, stopped having a secure job. From that point, my parents struggled to retain, mostly through debt, the markers of our "lower-middle-class" identity. I have opted to present myself as a working-class Mexican to avoid misrepresentation for the reader, especially if they are from countries where social class is less based on perception than on actual income, access to services and the right to leisure. For an interesting discussion of class in neo-liberal Mexico, see Cahn (2008).

26 For a discussion on what makes food to be considered as "traditional" and the problematics of this idea, see Sébastia (2017).

27 Porter (1995) offers an eloquent description of how objectivity and rigour came to be at the forefront in science and the social sciences and in the making of government decisions.

References

Abel, C., & Lewis, C. M. (eds.). (1985). *Latin America, economic imperialism and the state: The political economy of the external connection from independence to the present.* Bloomsbury Academic.

Abrantes Pêgo, R. (2010). *Salubristas y neosalubristas en la reforma del Estado: Grupos de interés en México e instituciones públicas de salud, 1982–2000 [The rise of the new public health: Neoliberal reforms and stakeholders in Mexico, 1982–2000]*. El Colegio de Michoacán.

Abu-Lughod, L. (1991). Writing against culture. In R. G. Fox (ed.), *Recapturing anthropology: Working in the present* (pp. 466–479). School of American Research Press.

Acuerdo Nacional para la Salud Alimentaria. Estrategia contra el sobrepeso y la obesidad [National Agreement for Nutritional Health. Strategy against overweight and obesity] (ANSA) (2010). Secretaría de Salud, México.

Agamben, G. (2009). *What is an apparatus? And other essays.* Stanford University Press.

Aguilar-Rivera, N., Rodríguez Lagunes, D. A., Enríquez Ruvalcaba, V., Castillo Morán, A., & Herrera Solano, A. (2012). The Mexican sugarcane industry: Overview, constraints, current status and long-term trends. *Sugar Tech,* 14(3), 207–222. https://doi.org/10.1007/s12355-012-0151-3.

Aguilar-Solís, S. (2006). *Iniciativa de decreto que reforma y adiciona diversas disposiciones de la Ley General de Salud [Proposal to reform the Health General Law]*. http://gaceta.dip utados.gob.mx/Gaceta/60/2006/dic/20061212-II.html.

Appadurai, A. (1981). Gastro-politics in Hindu South Asia. *American Ethnologist,* 8(3), 494–511. http://www.jstor.org/stable/644298.

Aradau, C., & Van Munster, R. (2007). Governing terrorism through risk: Taking precautions, (un)knowing the future. *European Journal of International Relations,* 13(1), 89–115. https://doi.org/10.1177/1354066107074290.

Ascencio Ramos, A. P. (2019). *Everyday experiences of women in mass-produced housing in the Metropolitan Area of Guadalajara, Mexico* [PhD, Carleton University].

Atkin, D., Faber, B., & González-Navarro, M. (2018). Retail globalization and household welfare: Evidence from Mexico. *Journal of Political Economy,* 126(1), 1–73. https://doi.org/10.1086/695476.

Babb, S. L. (2001). *Managing Mexico: Economists from nationalism to neoliberalism.* Princeton University Press. https://books.google.com.au/books?id=dkoVCvyqoo0C.

Baker, P., Machado, P., Santos, T., Sievert, K., Backholer, K., Hadjikakou, M., … Lawrence, M. (2020). Ultra-processed foods and the nutrition transition: Global, regional and national trends, food systems transformations and political economy drivers. *Obesity Reviews*, 21(12), e13126. https://doi.org/10.1111/obr.13126.

Banco de México (2022). *Balance of payments. Remittances.* https://www.banxico.org.mx/SieInternet/consultarDirectorioInternetAction.do?accion=consultarSeries.

Biles, J. J. (2006). Globalization of food retailing and the consequences of Wal-Martization in Mexico. In S. D. Brunn (ed.), *Wal-Mart world: The world's biggest corporation in the global economy* (pp. 343–356). Routledge.

Biltekoff, C. (2007). The terror within: Obesity in post 9/11 U.S. life. *American Studies*, 48(3), 29–48.

Blanes i Vidal, J., Draca, M., & Fons-Rosen, C. (2012). Revolving door lobbyists. *The American Economic Review*, 102(7), 3731–3748. http://dx.doi.org/10.1257/aer.102.7.3731.

Bonvecchio-Arenas, A., Theodore, F., Hernández-Cordero, S., Campirano-Núñez, F., Islas, A., Safdie, M., & Rivera-Dommarco, J. (2010). La Escuela como Alternativa en la Prevención de la Obesidad: La Experiencia en el Sistema Escolar Mexicano [The school as an opportunity for obesity prevention: An experience from the Mexican school system]. *Revista Española de Nutrición Comunitaria*, 16(1), 13–16. https://doi.org/10.1016/S1135-3074(10)70005–70003.

Brigg, M. (2001). Empowering NGOs: The microcredit movement through Foucault's notion of dispositif. Alternatives, 26(3), 233–258. https://doi.org/10.1177/030437540102600301.

Burchell, G. (2006). Translator's note. In M. Foucault (ed.), *Psychiatric power: Lectures at the Collège de France 1973–1974* (pp. xxii–xxiii). Palgrave Macmillan.

Bussolini, J. (2010). What is a dispositive? *Foucault Studies*, 10, 85–107.

Cahn, P. S. (2008). Consuming class: Multilevel marketers in neoliberal Mexico. *Cultural Anthropology*, 23(3), 429–452. https://doi.org/10.1111/j.1548-1360.2008.00014.x.

Centeno, M. A., & Maxfield, S. (1992). The marriage of finance and order: Changes in the Mexican political elite. *Journal of Latin American Studies*, 24(1), 57–85. http://doi.org/10.1017/S0022216X00022951.

Chandler, A., & Mazlish, B. (2005). Introduction. In A. Chandler & B. Mazlish (eds.), *Leviathans: Multinational corporations and the new global history* (pp. 1–16). Cambridge University Press. https://doi.org/10.1017/CBO9780511512025.

Chavez, M. (2002). The transformation of Mexican retailing with NAFTA. *Development Policy Review*, 20(4), 503–513. https://doi.org/10.1111/1467-7679.00186.

Clark, S. E., Hawkes, C., Murphy, S. M. E., Hansen-Kuhn, K. A., & Wallinga, D. (2012). Exporting obesity: US farm and trade policy and the transformation of the Mexican consumer food environment. *International Journal of Occupational and Environmental Health*, 18(1), 53–64. https://doi.org/10.1179/1077352512Z.0000000007.

CONADE (2014). *El programa Ponte al 100 [Ponte al 100 program]*. Retrieved August 29 from http://www.ponteal100.com/programa-ponte-al-100/.

Dallorso, N. S. (2012). Notas sobre el uso del Concepto de Dispositivo para el Análisis de Programas Sociales [Notes on the use of dispositif for the analysis of social programs]. *Espiral*, 19(54), 43–74. https://dialnet.unirioja.es/servlet/articulo?codigo=5345547.

De Janvry, A., Sadoulet, E., & Gordillo de Anda, G. (1995). NAFTA and Mexico's maize producers. *World Development*, 23(8), 1349–1362. https://doi.org/10.1016/0305-750X (95)00056-I.

Del Ángel-Pérez, A. L., & Rebolledo-Martínez, A. (2009). Familia, remesas y redes sociales en torno a la migración en Veracruz central [Family, remittances and migration networks from central Veracruz]. *Estudios fronterizos*, 10(19), 9–48. http://www.scielo.org.mx/scielo.php?script=sci_arttext&pid=S0187-69612009000100001&lng=es&nrm=iso&tlng=es.

Deleuze, G. (1992). What is a dispositif? In T. J. Armstrong (ed.), *Michel Foucault: Philosopher* (pp. 159–168). Routledge.

Delgado Wise, R., & Cypher, J. M. (2007). The strategic role of Mexican labor under NAFTA: Critical perspectives on current economic integration. *The Annals of the American Academy of Political and Social Science*, 610(1), 120–142. https://doi.org/10.1177/0002716206297527.

Denzin, N. K. (1998). The art and politics of interpretation. In Y. S. Lincoln & N. K. Denzin (eds.), *Collecting and interpreting qualitative materials* (pp. 313–344). Sage Publications.

Diario de los Debates [*Diary of debates*], Cámara de Diputados LX Legislatura (2007) (Año I, Segundo Periodo, 10 de abril de 2007). http://cronica.diputados.gob.mx/PDF/60/2007/abr/070410-2.pdf.

Diario de los Debates [*Diary of debates*], Cámara de Diputados LX Legislatura (2008) (Año II, Segundo Periodo, 17 de abril de 2008).

Dwyer, S. C., & Buckle, J. L. (2009). The space between: On being an insider–outsider in qualitative research. *International Journal of Qualitative Methods*, 8(1), 54–63. https://doi.org/10.1177/160940690900800105.

Escobar, A. (2011). *Encountering development: The making and unmaking of the third world* (2nd ed.). Princeton University Press.

Estevez, D. (2016, May 16). Remittances supersede oil as Mexico's main source of foreign exchange. *Forbes*. https://www.forbes.com/sites/doliaestevez/2016/05/16/remittances-supersede-oil-as-mexicos-main-source-of-foreign-income/?sh=74996b4a1754.

Estrategia Nacional para la Prevención y el Control del Sobrepeso, la Obesidad y la Diabetes [*National Strategy for the Prevention and Control of Overweight, Obesity and Diabetes*] *(ENSOD)* (2013). Secretaría de Salud, México.

Ferguson, J. (1990). *The anti-politics machine: "Development", depoliticization and bureaucratic power in Lesotho*. Cambridge University Press.

Flegal, K. M. (2022). How body size became a disease: A history of the Body Mass Index and its rise to clinical importance. In M. Gard, D. Powell, & J. Tenorio (eds.), *Routledge handbook of critical obesity studies* (pp. 23–39). Routledge.

Flegal, K. M., Graubard, B. I., Williamson, D. F., & Gail, M. H. (2005). Excess deaths associated with underweight, overweight, and obesity. *JAMA*, 293(15), 1861–1867. https://doi.org/10.1001/jama.293.15.1861.

Flegal, K. M., Ioannidis, J. P. A., & Doehner, W. (2019). Flawed methods and inappropriate conclusions for health policy on overweight and obesity: The Global BMI Mortality Collaboration meta-analysis. *Journal of Cachexia, Sarcopenia and Muscle*, 10 (1), 9–13. https://doi.org/10.1002/jcsm.12378.

Foley, M. W. (1995). Privatizing the countryside: The Mexican peasant movement and neoliberal reform. *Latin American Perspectives*, 22(1), 59–76. https://doi.org/10.1177/0094582x9502200105.

Foucault, M. (1980). *Power/knowledge: Selected interviews and other Writings 1972–1977*, edited by C. Gordon, L. Marshall, J. Mepham, & K. Soper; translated by C. Gordon. Pantheon Books.

Foucault, M. (2008). *The birth of biopolitics: Lectures at the Collège De France 1978–1979*, translated by G. Burchell. Picador.

Fox, J. (1992). *The politics of food in Mexico: State power and social mobilization*. Cornell University Press.

Fox, J., & Hernández, L. (1992). Mexico's difficult democracy: Grassroots movements, NGOs, and local government. *Alternatives: Global, Local, Political*, 17(2), 165–208. http://www.jstor.org/stable/40644738.

Fuentes, F. (2007, June 22). Fundación Mídete inicia guerra contra obesidad [Mídete Foundation starts war against obesity]. *El Universal*. https://archivo.eluniversal.com.mx/articulos/40853.html.

Fundación Coca-Cola (n.d.). *Ponte al 100*. Retrieved August 25 from http://fundacion coca-cola.com.mx/programas/ponte_al_100.html.

FUNSALUD (ed.). (1994). *Nutrición clínica 1994* [*Clinical nutrition 1994*]. Editorial Médica Panamericana.

FUNSALUD (n.d.). FUNSALUD. http://funsalud.org.mx/funsalud/.

Gaddis, J. E. (2020). *The labor of lunch: Why we need real food and real jobs in American public schools.* University of California Press.

Gálvez, A. (2018). *Eating NAFTA: Trade, food policies, and the destruction of Mexico.* University of California Press.

Gard, M. (2010). *The end of the obesity epidemic.* Routledge.

Gard, M., Powell, D., & Tenorio, J. (eds.). (2022). *Routledge handbook of critical obesity studies.* Routledge. https://doi.org/10.4324/9780429344824.

Gard, M., & Wright, J. (2005). *Obesity epidemic: Science, morality and ideology.* Routledge.

Gochman, B. P. (1998). *Networks, neoliberalism, and NAFTA: Economic technocrats and policy change in Mexico, 1982–1997* [PhD, University of Denver].

Gómez, E. J. (2019). Coca-Cola's political and policy influence in Mexico: understanding the role of institutions, interests and divided society. *Health Policy and Planning*, 34(7), 520–528. https://doi.org/10.1093/heapol/czz063.

Greenhalgh, S. (2012). Weighty subjects: The biopolitics of the U.S. war on fat. *American Ethnologist*, 39(3), 471–487. https://doi.org/10.1111/j.1548-1425.2012.01375.x.

Greenhalgh, S. (2021). Inside ILSI: How Coca-Cola, working through its scientific non-profit, created a global science of exercise for obesity and got it embedded in Chinese policy (1995–2015). *Journal of Health Politics, Policy and Law*, 46(2), 235–276. https://doi.org/10.1215/03616878-8802174.

Guthman, J. (2008). Bringing good food to others: Investigating the subjects of alternative food practice. *Cultural Geographies*, 15(4), 431–447.

Guthman, J. (2022). Obesity and its cures as socio-ecological fixes for agro-food capitalism. In M. Gard, D. Powell, & J. Tenorio (eds.), *Routledge handbook of critical obesity studies* (pp. 135–143). Routledge.

Harner, J., Jiménez Huerta, E., & Cruz Solís, H. (2009). Buying development: Housing and urban growth in Guadalajara, Mexico. *Urban Geography*, 30(5), 465–489. https://doi.org/10.2747/0272-3638.30.5.465.

Hawkes, C. (2002). Marketing activities of global soft drink and fast food companies in emerging markets: A review. In *Globalization, diets and noncommunicable diseases*. World Health Organization. https://apps.who.int/iris/bitstream/handle/10665/42609/9241590416.pdf;sequence=1.

Hawkes, C. (2006). Uneven dietary development: Linking the policies and processes of globalization with the nutrition transition, obesity and diet-related chronic diseases. *Globalization and Health*, 2(1), 4. https://doi.org/10.1186/1744-8603-2-4.

Herrick, C. (2009). Shifting blame/selling health: Corporate social responsibility in the age of obesity. *Sociology of Health & Illness*, 31(1), 51–65. https://doi.org/10.1111/j.1467-9566.2008.01121.x.

Howell, J., & Ingham, A. (2001). From social problem to personal issue: The language of lifestyle. *Cultural Studies*, 15(2), 326–351. https://doi.org/10.1080/09502380152390535.

Inclán Valadez, M. C. (2013). *The 'Casas GEO' movement: An ethnography of a new housing experience in Cuernavaca, Mexico* [PhD, The London School of Economics and Political Science].

INEGI (2021). *Conociendo la industria del chocolate y la confitería* [*Exploring the confectionery and chocolate industry in Mexico*], Colección de Estudios Sectorial y Regionales. https://www.inegi.org.mx/contenidos/productos/prod_serv/contenidos/espanol/bvinegi/productos/nueva_estruc/889463902409.pdf.

Ingham, A. G. (1985). From public issue to personal trouble: Well-being and the fiscal crisis of the state. *Sociology of Sport Journal*, 2(1), 43. https://doi.org/10.1123/ssj.2.1.43.

Jenatton, M., & Morales, H. (2020). Civilized cola and peasant pozol: Young people's social representations of a traditional maize beverage and soft drinks within food systems of Chiapas, Mexico. *Agroecology and Sustainable Food Systems*, 44(8), 1052–1088. https://doi.org/10.1080/21683565.2019.1631935.

Lather, P. (1993). Fertile obsession: Validity after poststructuralism. *The Sociological Quarterly*, 34(4), 673–693. http://www.jstor.org/stable/4121374.

Laurell, A. C. (2012). La [sic] regreso de Funsalud [The return of Funsalud]. *La Jornada*. https://www.jornada.com.mx/2012/12/07/opinion/a03a1cie.

Laurell, A. C. (2015a). The Mexican Popular Health Insurance: Myths and realities. *International Journal of Health Services*, 45(1), 105–124. https://doi.org/10.2190/HS.45.1.h.

Laurell, A. C. (2015b). Three decades of neoliberalism in Mexico: The destruction of society. *International Journal of Health Services*, 45(2), 246–264. https://doi.org/10.1177/0020731414568507.

Leatherman, T. L., & Goodman, A. (2005). Coca-colonization of diets in the Yucatan. *Social Science & Medicine*, 61(4), 833–846. https://doi.org/10.1016/j.socscimed.2004.08.047.

Levine, S. (2008). *School lunch politics: The surprising history of America's favorite welfare program*. Princeton University Press.

Li, T. M. (2007). Practices of assemblage and community forest management. *Economy and Society*, 36(2), 263–293. http://doi.org/10.1080/03085140701254308.

Lineamientos 2010 (Acuerdo mediante el cual se establecen los lineamientos generales para el expendio o distribución de alimentos y bebidas en los establecimientos de consumo escolar de los planteles de educación básica [General guidelines for the distribution or sales of food and drinks by retailers within basic education schools]) (2010). Diario Oficial de la Federación: Órgano del Gobierno Constitucional de los Estados Unidos Mexicanos.

Lineamientos 2014 (Acuerdo mediante el cual se establecen los lineamientos generales para el expendio y distribución de alimentos y bebidas preparados y procesados en las escuelas del Sistema Educativo Nacional [Guidelines for the sales and distribution of prepared and processed food and drinks in the Mexican national education system]) (2014). Diario Oficial de la Federación: Órgano del Gobierno Constitucional de los Estados Unidos Mexicanos.

Lougheed, T. (2006). Policy: WHO/ILSI affiliation sustained. *Environmental Health Perspectives*, 114(9), A521–A521. https://doi.org/doi:10.1289/ehp.114-a521a.

Marcus, G. E. (1995). Ethnography in/of the world system: The emergence of multi-sited ethnography. *Annual Review of Anthropology*, 24(1), 95–117. https://doi.org/10.1146/annurev.an.24.100195.000523.

Mazari-Hiriart, M., Espinosa, A. C., López-Vidal, Y., Arredondo-Hernández, R., Díaz-Torres, E., & Equihua-Zamora, C. (2010). Visión integral sobre el agua y la salud [A holistic approach to the relation between water and health]. In B. Jiménez-Cisneros, M. L. Torregrosa y Armentia, & L. Aboites-Aguilar (eds.), *El agua en México: Cauces y encauces* (pp. 291–315). Academia Mexicana de Ciencias.

Mejía-Haro, A., & Corichi-García, S. (2007). *Proyecto de decreto por el que se adiciona una fracción IX al artículo 115 y un párrafo tercero al artículo 216 de la Ley General de Salud* [*Draft decree adding a section IX to article 115 and a third paragraph to article 216 of the General Health Law*]. https://www.senado.gob.mx/64/gaceta_del_senado/documento/15001.

Mialon, M., & Gomes, F. d. S. (2019). Public health and the ultra-processed food and drink products industry: Corporate political activity of major transnationals in Latin America and the Caribbean. *Public Health Nutrition*, 22(10), 1898–1908. https://doi.org/10.1017/S1368980019000417.

Mialon, M., Ho, M., Carriedo, A., Ruskin, G., & Crosbie, E. (2021). Beyond nutrition and physical activity: food industry shaping of the very principles of scientific integrity. *Globalization and Health*, 17(1), 37. https://doi.org/10.1186/s12992-021-00689-1.

Monteiro, C. A. (2009). Nutrition and health. The issue is not food, nor nutrients, so much as processing. *Public Health Nutrition*, 12(5), 729–731. https://doi.org/10.1017/S1368980009005291.

Monteiro, C. A., Levy, R. B., Claro, R. M., Ribeiro de Castro, I. R., & Cannon, G. (2010). A new classification of foods based on the extent and purpose of their processing. *Cadernos de Saúde Pública*, 26(11), 2039–2049.

Montero García, L. A., & Thébout, V. (2018). *Veracruz, tierra de cañaverales: Grupos sociales, conflictos y dinámicas de expansión*. Instituto Nacional de Antropología e Historia.

Montes de Oca-Barrera, L. B. (2018). *Comida chatarra: Entre la gobernanza regulatioria y la simulación* [*Junk food: Between governance and simulation*]. Universidad Nacional Autónoma de México.

Moodie, R., Bennett, E., Kwong, E. J. L., Santos, T. M., Pratiwi, L., Williams, J., & Baker, P. (2021). Ultra-processed profits: The political economy of countering the global spread of ultra-processed foods—a synthesis review on the market and political practices of transnational food corporations and strategic public health responses. *International Journal of Health Policy and Management*, 10 (Special Issue on Political Economy of Food Systems), 968–982. https://doi.org/10.34172/ijhpm.2021.45.

Morris, S. D. (1999). Corruption and the Mexican political system: Continuity and change. *Third World Quarterly*, 20(3), 623–643. https://doi.org/10.1080/01436599913721.

Morris, S. D. (2009). *Political corruption in Mexico: The impact of democratization*. Lynne Rienner Publishers.

Nash, J. (2007). Consuming interests: Water, rum, and Coca-Cola from ritual propitiation to corporate expropriation in highland Chiapas. *Cultural Anthropology*, 22(4), 621–639. https://doi.org/10.1525/can.2007.22.4.621.

Nava-Tablada, M. E. (2012). Migración internacional y caficultura en Veracruz, México. *Migraciones Internacionales*, 6(3), 139–171.

Navarro, V. (2007). Neoliberalism as a class ideology; Or, the political causes of the growth of inequalities. *International Journal of Health Services*, 37(1), 47–62. https://doi.org/10.2190/ap65-x154-4513-r520.

Nestle, M. (2015). *Soda politics: Taking on big soda (and winning)*. Oxford University Press.

Ochoa, R., & Pereyra, B. (2014). La mascarada de Ponte al 100 [The Ponte al 100 hoax]. *Proceso*. https://www.proceso.com.mx/382656/la-mascarada-de-ponte-al-100.

Olaiz-Fernández, G., Rivera-Dommarco, J., Shamah-Levy, T., Rojas, R., Villalpando-Hernández, S., Hernández-Avila, M., & Sepúlveda-Amor, J. (2006). *Encuesta Nacional de Salud y Nutrición 2006 [2006 Mexican National Health and Nutrition Survey]*. Instituto Nacional de Salud Pública.

Olvera, A. J. (2003). Las tendencias generales del desarrollo de la sociedad civil en México [General tendencies in the development of the civil society as a political actor in Mexico]. In A. J. Olvera (ed.), *Sociedad civil, esfera pública y democratización en América Latina: México [Civil society, public sphere and democratization in Latin America: Mexico]* (pp. 42–70). Universidad Veracruzana/Fondo de Cultura Económica.

Ong, A. (2007). Neoliberalism as a mobile technology. *Transactions of the Institute of British Geographers*, 32(1), 3–8. https://doi.org/10.1111/j.1475-5661.2007.00234.x.

Otero, G. (1996). Neoliberal reform and politics in Mexico: An overview. In G. Otero (ed.), *Neoliberalism revisited: Economic restructuring and Mexico's political future* (pp. 1–25). Westview Press.

Otero, G. (2011). Neoliberal globalization, NAFTA, and migration: Mexico's loss of food and labor sovereignty. *Journal of Poverty*, 15(4), 384–402. https://doi.org/10.1080/10875549.2011.614514.

Otero, G. (2018). *The neoliberal diet: Healthy profits, unhealthy people*. University of Texas Press.

Otero, G. (2021). The neoliberal diet. In A. H. Akram-Lodhi, K. Dietz, B. Engels, & B. M. McKay (eds.), *Handbook of critical agrarian studies* (pp. 556–560). Edward Elgar Publishing.

Otero, G., & Butler Flora, C. (2009). Sweet protectionism: State policy and employment in the sugar industries of the NAFTA countries. In J. M. Rivera, S. Whiteford, & M. Chávez (eds.), *NAFTA and the campesinos: The impact of NAFTA in small-scale agricultural producers in Mexico and the prospects for change* (pp. 63–88). University of Scranton Press.

Pastor, R. (1993). NAFTA as the center of an integration process: The nontrade issues. *The Brookings Review*, 11(1), 40–45. https://doi.org/10.2307/20080364.

Patel, R. (2009). *Stuffed and starved: Markets, power and the hidden battle for the world food system*. Black Inc.

Pereyra, B. (2014). Se desinfla Ponte al 100 [Ponte al 100 goes bad]. *Proceso*. https://www.proceso.com.mx/386780.

Pérez-Monterosas, M. (2012). "Nuevos" orígenes y "nuevos" destinos de la migración México-Estados Unidos: El caso del centro de Veracruz ["New" origins and "new" destinations in the Mexico-US migration: The case of Veracruz' central region]. *Espiral*, 19(54), 195–232.

Pilcher, J. M. (2004). Industrial tortillas and folkloric Pepsi: The nutritional consequences of hybrid cuisines in Mexico. In J. L. Watson & M. L. Caldwell (eds.), *The cultural politics of food and eating: A reader* (pp. 235–250). Wiley-Blackwell.

Pilcher, J. M. (2013). Taco Bell, Maseca, and Slow Food: A postmodern apocalypse for Mexico's peasant cuisine? In C. Counihan & P. Van Esterik (eds.), *Food and culture: A reader* (3rd ed., pp. 426–436). Routledge.

Plazas, M. (2010). Juego y Comida dan salud a tu vida [Eat and play make you healthy]. *Revista Latinoamericana de Estudios Educativos*, 40(2), 153–164. https://www.cee.edu.mx/rlee/revista/r2001_2010/r_texto/t_2010_2_07.pdf.

PODER (2016). *Funsalud, los empresarion que marcan las políticas de salud en México [Funsalud, how business groups shape health policy in Mexico]*. https://www.rindecuentas.

org/reportajes/2016/04/07/funsalud-los-empresarios-tras-las-politicas-de-salud/#
fnref-705-1.

Poppendieck, J. (2010). *Free for all: Fixing school food in America*. University of California
Press.

Porter, T. M. (1995). *Trust in numbers: The pursuit of objectivity in science and public life*.
Princeton University Press.

Powell, D. (2020). *Schools, corporations, and the war on childhood obesity: How corporate
philanthropy shapes public health and education*. Routledge.

Powell, D., Tenorio, J., & Gard, M. (2022). The worlds of critical obesity studies. In M.
Gard, D. Powell, & J. Tenorio (eds.), *Routledge handbook of critical obesity studies* (pp.
2–8). Routledge.

Reardon, T., & Berdegué, J. A. (2002). The rapid rise of supermarkets in Latin America:
Challenges and opportunities for development. *Development Policy Review*, 20(4), 371–
388. https://doi.org/10.1111/1467-7679.00178.

Reyes, A. (2020). Mexico's housing paradox: Tensions between financialization and
access. *Housing Policy Debate*, 30(4), 486–511. https://doi.org/10.1080/
10511482.2019.1709879.

Safdie, M., Jennings-Aburto, N., Levesque, L., Janssen, I., Campirano-Nunez, F., Lopez-
Olmedo, N., Aburto, T., & Rivera, J. A. (2013). Impact of a school-based intervention
program on obesity risk factors in Mexican children. *Salud Pública de México*, 55(3),
374–387.

Safdie, M., Lévesque, L., González-Casanova, I., Salvo, D., Islas, A., Hernández-Cordero,
S., Bonvecchio, A., & Rivera, J. A. (2013). Promoting healthful diet and physical activity
in the Mexican school system for the prevention of obesity in children. *Salud Pública de
México*, 55(3), s357–s373.

Saguy, A., & Riley, K. (2005). Weighing both sides: Morality, mortality, and framing
contests over obesity. *Journal of Health Politics, Policy and Law*, 20(5), 869–921. https://
doi.org/10.1215/03616878-30-5-869.

Sant'Anna, D. B. d. (2016). *Gordos, magros e obesos: Uma história do peso no Brasil* [*Fatness,
thinness and obesity: A history of bodies and weight in Brazil*]. Estação Liberdade.

Schwartz, H. (1986). *Never satisfied: A cultural history of diets, fantasies, and fat*. Anchor
Books.

Schwentesius, R., & Gómez, M. Á. (2002). Supermarkets in Mexico: Impacts on horti-
culture systems. *Development Policy Review*, 20(4), 487–502. https://doi.org/10.
1111/1467-7679.00185.

Scrinis, G. (2013). *Nutritionism: The science and politics of dietary advice*. Columbia University Press.

Scrinis, G. (2020). Ultra-processed foods and the corporate capture of nutrition—an essay
by Gyorgy Scrinis. *BMJ (Clinical Research ed.)*, 371, m4601. https://doi.org/10.
1136/bmj.m4601.

Sébastia, B. (2017). Eating traditional food: Politics, identity and practices. In B. Sébastia
(ed.), *Eating traditional food: Politics, identity and practices* (pp. 1–19). Routledge.

Sentíes-Herrera, H. E., Gómez-Merino, F. C., Valdez-Balero, A., Silva-Rojas, H. V., &
Trejo-Téllez, L. I. (2014). The agro-industrial sugarcane system in Mexico: Current
status, challenges and opportunities. *Journal of Agricultural Science*, 6(4), 26–54.

Shore, C., & Wright, S. (1997). Policy: A new field of anthropology. In C. Shore & S.
Wright (eds.), *Anthropology of policy: Critical perspectives on governance and power* (pp.
3–34). Routledge.

statista (2013). Annual per capita consumption of Coca-Cola's beverage products from 1991 to 2012, by country. https://www.statista.com/statistics/271156/per-capita-consumption-of-soft-drinks-of-the-coca-cola-company-by-country/.

Stearns, P. (1997). *Fat history: Bodies and beauty in the modern West.* New York University Press.

U.S.–Mexican Relations: Joint Statement by Presidents Bush and Salinas de Gortari. (1991). *Foreign Policy Bulletin*, 1(4–5), 134–136. doi:10.1017/S1052703600008728. https://www.cambridge.org/core/journals/foreign-policy-bulletin/article/abs/usm exican-relations-joint-statement-by-presidents-bush-and-salinas-de-gortari/046923DF 15001E7251C10F571674CE19.

USDA (2014). *Processed product spotlight: Confectionery* [International Agricultural Trade Report.]. Foreign Agricultural Service—United States Department of Agriculture. https://www.fas.usda.gov/sites/default/files/2015-02/confectionery_iatr_march_2014.pdf.

Valdés Ugalde, F. (1997). *Autonomía y legitimidad: los empresarios, la política y el estado en México [Autonomy and legitimacy: Businessmen, politics and the Mexican state].* Siglo XXI Editores.

Wise, T. A. (2009). *Agricultural dumping under NAFTA: Estimating the costs of U.S. agricultural policies to Mexican producers.* Working paper (09–08), Global Development and Environment Institute, 1–38. https://ageconsearch.umn.edu/record/179078.

Yunez-Naude, A., & Barceinas Paredes, F. (2002). *Lessons from NAFTA: The case of Mexico's agricultural sector.* Final Report to the World Bank. http://ctrc.sice.oas.org/geo graph/north/yunez.pdf.

Zahniser, S., & Coyle, W. (2004). *U.S.–Mexico corn trade during the NAFTA era: New twists to an old story* (FDS-04D-01). Economic Research Service USDA. https://www.ers.usda.gov/webdocs/outlooks/36451/49338_fds04d01.pdf?v=374.2.

2 Food, Public Health and Education in the Making of Mexico

Portraits of Enrique Peña Nieto, the Mexican President (2012–2018), hung on the walls of most government spaces I visited during my fieldwork. At Benito Juárez Primary School, paintings of Peña Nieto and Javier Duarte, the Governor of Veracruz (2010–2016), both from the Partido Revolucionario Institucional (PRI), were displayed in the office of the principal, Susana. I appreciated their symbolism. During my years working in education in Veracruz, I learned that the presence, or absence, of portraits usually suggested principals' implied support for a party. As my sources put it, Susana was well "connected" with the ruling party. During our casual conversations Susana reinforced this point, emphasizing how her "contacts", friends in state government positions, had helped the school many times. "The party that does the most for the school will attract more votes from the parents", she said as she explained to me the importance of asking for support during elections.

Unsurprisingly, the construction of a dining room and kitchen for Benito Juárez Primary School started in May 2016, four weeks before the elections for the state governor. Funding came from a federal school infrastructure program whose targets were rural, under-resourced schools. In the lead-up to elections, however, the state government relocated the funds to schools in key electoral districts, regardless of whether they met the program's selection criteria. At the time of my fieldwork, Veracruz had been ruled by the PRI since 1929, when the party was created, but after more than 80 years in power, the PRI was ranking second in the 2016 state-election polls. The electoral district where Benito Juárez Primary School was located was the largest in the state, and the second largest in the country: the PRI could not afford to lose it (for the key role teachers play in political processes in Mexico, see Larreguy et al., 2017).

In terms of infrastructure and services, Benito Juárez Primary School was exceedingly well-resourced, far beyond the average urban public school in Veracruz. The school already had an equipped kitchen, but the new construction would give parents the impression that the government was doing something for them. This is one of multiple examples of the political uses of policy in Mexico, which gives a particular flavor to the construction and deployment of 'healthy lifestyles'. The political use of policy is, like probably anywhere else around the world, not new in Mexico. From its creation, the PRI, which ruled for 70 years

DOI: 10.4324/9781003356264-2

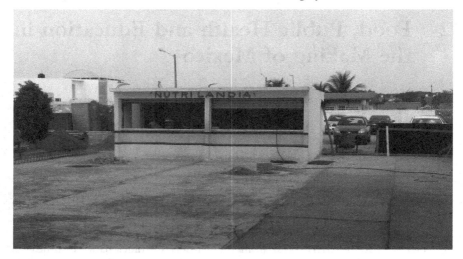

Figure 2.1 Renovations underway at "Nutrilandia"—the cooperativa escolar at Benito
    Juárez Primary School—in May 2016. Photo by the author.

between 1929 and 2000, had direct control of and mobilized unions for political
purposes. Education authorities and teachers were not exempt. Schools, food and
public health have historically been a vehicle to expand projects of government.
Therefore, I find it compelling to explain how the forms the Mexican state has
taken from the early twentieth century and how education, food and public health
policy have been used to manage the population.

In this chapter, I offer the reader a contextualization of Mexican politics that is
central to my analysis. History helps us to understand why the regulation of school
food practices in the name of health became an imperative from the mid-2000s
and became even more significant after 2010. My goal with this history is to
broaden the current discussion that presents schools as "anti-obesity sites" and
"obesogenic environments", without acknowledging the complex politics that
have historically surrounded policy implementation in schools.

This chapter is divided into three sections. In the first section, I offer a general
overview of Mexican politics through the twentieth century. This section is
intended to provide the reader with information about how a shift in government
and economic practices enabled the transition of Mexico from a "corporatist" to a
"neoliberal" state. For this reason, I describe how the PRI was created and the
political changes that this party, and Mexico, experienced through the century. I
have structured this section mainly around the PRI because one cannot claim to
understand Mexican politics and policy implementation without knowing the origins, evolution, contradictions and contributions of this party. Drawing on this
general history of Mexican politics, in the second section, I describe how Mexican
policymakers of the first half of the twentieth century used education and food
policy to construct a 'modern' population and to enlarge the corporatist state.[1]
Furthermore, I show how public health policy in Mexico has been influenced, to

some extent, by the interests of the United States and, since the 1980s, shaped by a group of "free-market enthusiasts" managing the health sector. In the last section, I use the previous sections as a backdrop to explain how school food regulations changed from a "cooperative" to a "healthy lifestyles" model.

From Corporativism to Neoliberalism: Forms of Government in Twentieth Century Mexico

In the autumn of 1910, popular discontent against the dictatorship of Porfirio Díaz, who had ruled Mexico for more than 30 years, triggered the Mexican Revolution. The revolution was a multifaceted event where multiple groups, agendas and ideals were at play between 1910 and 1929 (for an example of the diversity of interests, see Smith, 2015). Historians have offered multiple readings of the nature, scope, effects and timing of the revolution (for two different interpretations, see Knight, 1985 and Ruíz, 1982). For instance, in terms of timing, there is disagreement about when the revolution came to an end. For some scholars, the promulgation of the Constitution of 1917 marked the culmination of the revolution, whereas for others the revolution finished when Álvaro Obregón (1920–1924) became president of Mexico in 1920. In other cases, historians have argued that the revolution ended in 1929, when Plutarco Elías Calles,[2] a wealthy revolutionary general from northern Mexico and an influential secretary of interior during the Obregón administration, founded the Partido Nacional Revolucionario (PNR) (Knight, 2010). For the purposes of this discussion, I consider that the formation of the PNR contributed to ending the armed conflict, enabling the political conditions to engineer the bases of the Mexican state.[3]

Calles was in office from 1924–1928 but remained Mexico's central political figure into the early 1930s. Using his vast political capital and influence, Calles was able to reconcile divergent political factions and group them under the PNR in March 1929. Between 1928 and 1934, he selected four consecutive presidential candidates which, according to some historians, allowed him to remain the "power behind the scenes" (Buchenau, 2006, p. 144). In 1934, Lázaro Cárdenas, another revolutionary general, won the presidential election with the support of Calles. Unlike his predecessors, however, Cárdenas did not comply with Calles' rule and, during his first year of government, initiated a series of political moves to cut Calles out of political power. The Calles–Cárdenas break up was finalized in April 1936, when Calles was sent into exile.

Cárdenas pursued a nationalist and socialist-oriented plan of government. He initiated an agrarian reform, adopted a nationalist economic policy which resulted in the expropriation of the oil industry, and used social policy to reduce the increasing social unrest. Cárdenas also accelerated the transformation of the rural Mexican population into a large workforce that would feed the growing industrialization of the country. For this purpose, as I describe below, a large educational campaign was launched.

Under the Cárdenas administration, the Mexican state was developed according to a corporatist perspective (for an extended discussion on the conceptualization of corporatism, see Schmitter, 1974). In this form of government, the state has a central role in the management of the economy and the organization and structure of the political system. Cárdenas' government has been considered as corporatist, as Weston (1983) explains, for the way in which he created and mobilized different groups under the organization of the PNR. Before Cárdenas took on both the Mexican presidency and control of the PNR, the party had been controlled by the military and leaders representing the middle class. He pushed to group workers and peasants into state-controlled mass organizations, which at the same time granted him with wide political power to transform the PNR from a "party of generals and regional strongmen" into "an 'inclusionary corporatist' mass party" (Fox, 1992, p. 47). Then, in 1938, with vast popular support from the mass organizations of workers and peasants, Cárdenas reorganized the PNR and changed its name to the Partido de la Revolución Mexicana (PRM). These mass organizations and the nascent unions, the teachers' union among them, had a pivotal role in Cárdenas' corporatist project. The bases of the corporatist state established by Cárdenas in the 1930s were expanded by his successors. Nevertheless, they moved away from the socialist flavor of Cárdenas' policies.

Supported by Cárdenas, Manuel Ávila Camacho[4] effortlessly won the 1940 presidential elections. Gónzalez Casanova (1986, p. 123) argues that Ávila Camacho used the corporatist organization of the state inherited from his successor, but also refurbished old "revolutionary symbols and discourses" with the aim of developing a "new *form of government*".[5] This paradigm shift in government materialized in the change of the party's name. In January 1946, in the last year of Ávila Camacho's term, the PRM changed its name to the current PRI. Historians of Mexican politics have claimed that this event expressed the power of the new political elite which would rule the PRI, and Mexico, as represented by the then-presidential candidate, and eventually president of Mexico, Miguel Alemán (Gónzalez Casanova, 1986; Garrido, 1991).

In spite of the internal struggles, the so-called "party of the revolution" brought a certain level of "political stability" to Mexico between the 1940s and the late-1970s. In contrast to its neighbors in Latin America or other countries from the Third World,[6] Mexico did not experience a military dictatorship during the twentieth century. In a not-so-democratic way, however, the president directly designated his successor, usually the person serving as secretary of interior, which resulted in smooth presidential transitions. According to Smith (2015), the political stability together with nationalist economic policies created the conditions for accelerated economic growth, or what has been considered the "Mexican Miracle".

The rapid economic growth between the 1940s and the 1960s, known as the "Mexican Miracle", significantly enlarged the middle class and strengthened the purchasing power of some working-class sectors (for a critique, see Carmona et al., 1970). However, the so-called "Miracle" was not experienced by all Mexicans (Ford, 2008; Lewis, 1959, 1961; Schryer, 2014).[7] Furthermore, the alleged political stability that enabled the "Mexican Miracle" was not achieved magically. Scholars of Mexico in the second half of the twentieth century, for instance, have documented how political dissidents were usually repressed by PRI governments (Pensado, 2013; Sherman, 2000) and how this party used food policy to keep popular discontent within a manageable margin, especially in the emerging large urban areas where the PRI's popularity had started to decrease (Fox, 1992; Ochoa, 2002). To maintain the political system under the party's rule, the PRI closely dominated workers' organizations. Morales-Gómez and Torres (1990) claim that between the 1950s and 1970s, the state allocated significant resources to public education in order to have the teachers' unions as a political arm at the service of the PRI.

Economic growth enabled different practices of corruption at all levels of government, which allowed people connected with the party to benefit at the expense of others. Garrido (1991) comments that from the 1940s, public servants and union leaders took illegal advantage of Mexico's increasing industrial growth to become wealthy. High-level government officials and the Mexican presidents themselves also stole public funds to increase their personal and familial wealth (Knight, 1996; Morris, 1999; Niblo, 1999).

Corruption, Lomnitz (2001) claims, has been present in Mexican politics since the colonial era. However, some scholars have argued that it was in the mid-1940s, under the presidency of Miguel Alemán, that political corruption became widespread (Morris, 1999) and reached stunning proportions (Niblo, 1999; Sherman, 2000). In 1946, Alemán became the first non-military president after the revolution. He abandoned many of the social reforms that his predecessors had begun and favored private and foreign investment to bolster national industries that lacked capital. These actions contributed, to some extent, to the Mexican economic boom. Nonetheless, many scholars have argued that most of Alemán's decisions were taken with the aim of creating profits for himself and his friends (Bunker & Macías-González, 2011; Joseph & Buchenau, 2013; Pérez Monfort, 2011). Seeking personal benefits became a kind of rule for government officials during the years of economic bonanza.

In 1963, Mexico's bid for the 1968 Olympics was successful. Mexico was now seen as being in the position to host such an important event. For the first time, a Third World country would host the Olympics. Nonetheless, 1968 was a year of contrasts in Mexico. On 12 October, the Olympics were inaugurated in Mexico City, showing the world an image of the 'modern' Mexico and its ongoing process of development (Zolov, 2004). But a few days before, on 2 October, thousands of students, who had been demonstrating for democracy, were repressed during a rally. According to Pensado (2013, p. 2), hundreds of these students were "ambushed and brutally killed or arrested by government authorities". After this event, as some historians have argued (Walker, 2013), the "Mexican Miracle" started to vanish.

The corporatist state increased its use of force to control social upheaval. In 1970, Luis Echeverría was elected president. Having been the secretary of interior from 1964 to 1970, he was seen as one of the government officials most responsible for the students' repression (Sherman, 2000), and that election showed a clear decrease in the PRI's popular support. Spalding (1981) argues that the PRI's loss of popular support and dominance over workers organizations increased tensions between the state and the private sector. Mexicans woke up from the dream as the country entered a deep economic crisis in the late 1970s and early 1980s. Dramatic shifts in politics and policy were about to come, together with an entire new form of government.

From the creation of the PRI in the late 1920s until the 1970s, the PRI and the Mexican state coexisted almost as one entity, which, amongst other reasons, is why Mexico was considered a corporatist state (for a critique, see Rubin, 1996). After his election in 1970, Echeverría was the last president who served as the secretary of interior in the previous administration. After 1975, the PRI's presidial candidates who were selected had served either within the treasury or the budgeting and planning secretariats (Camp, 2011). This minor change in the selection criterion of presidential candidates sheds some light on the political and economic transformations that Mexico experienced after 1980.

In political terms, during the 1980s a new breed of politicians became the dominant group within the PRI. The "political technocrats", as Camp (1985) calls them, radically transformed the form of government that the party had pursued since its formation, including the many changes I have discussed here. Although he contends that "technocrats" had been part of Mexican politics before the 1980s, Camp (1985, p. 108) also argues that Miguel de la Madrid, president from 1982 to 1988, epitomized "the ascension to control of the new Mexican administrative elite".[8] According to Camp and other researchers' studies on technocrats in Mexico (Babb, 2001; Centeno & Maxfield, 1992), this new political elite dominating the PRI was different from their fellow party members in two ways. First, they had been trained in economics in elite US universities and, second, they did not require popular support to occupy government posts. What mattered most was technical economic knowledge, efficiency, fluency in English and a well-developed national and international network.

The Mexican economy also experienced a radical transformation in the 1980s. Affected by a deep economic crisis early in the decade, Mexico was asked by the International Monetary Fund and the World Bank to implement a set of structural adjustment policies to limit state intervention and to open the economy to the global market (Stallings, 1992). According to various scholars, these events marked the start of the "neoliberal" era in Mexico (Babb, 2001; Laurell, 2015b; Otero, 1996; Pastor & Wise, 1997). The rise of the technocrats and the "neoliberalization" of Mexico occurred concurrently. President De la Madrid and his team of "cosmopolitan, well-travelled economic technocrats", as Gochman (1998, p. 85) has argued, started to dismantle the corporatist state and lay the foundations for a neoliberal Mexican government. However, as Camp (2011, p. 474) claims, while the technocrats were significantly transforming the economy, they did not see "an immediate need for altering the Mexican political model, [or for] making both the model and their party structure more democratic". Instead, corruption kept growing (Gochman, 1998).

In 1988, Carlos Salinas, an economist with a Master's and a PhD from Harvard, became president (1988–1994) in a highly controversial election (Magaloni,

2008). He privatized public companies and reversed Cárdenas' agrarian reform. Salinas used social policy to "shift power away from traditional, clientelist sources toward more technocratic-oriented decision-makers" (Morris, 2009, p. 11). His aim was to advance neoliberalism beyond its economic dimensions and establish what can be called a *neoliberal form of government* in Mexico. Salinas was *the* architect of NAFTA (Pastor, 1993), which was signed in 1994 to liberate commerce and reduce, or eliminate in other cases, import tariffs between Mexico, the USA and Canada.

After 70 years of ruling Mexico, the PRI was defeated in the 2000 presidential election. According to some scholars (Baer, 2004; Klesner, 2001), influenced by increasing popular unrest against corruption from successive PRI governments and the escalating uneven distribution of wealth, Mexicans elected the right-wing candidate Vicente Fox from the Partido Acción Nacional (PAN). There were great expectations of change. Although he led some improvements towards democracy, Fox's presidency ultimately failed to meet popular expectations. Pastor and Wise (2005) have claimed that the Fox administration did not achieve great improvements due to his team's lack of "political skills". Fox recruited much of his government personnel from the private sector. Consequently, if the PRI technocrats had facilitated corporate expansion, Fox's administration legitimized the "private sector's open role in politics" (Camp, 2008, p. 303). Having been the Director of Coca-Cola Mexico, Vicente Fox, according to scholars from a range of fields (Ballinas & Méndez, 2006; Caldera Ortega, 2017; Delgado-Ramos, 2014; Nash, 2007), worked to consolidate the power of corporations and pursued an agenda that prioritized private interests. As I show in Chapter 6, Fox was instrumental in the expansion of the bottled water market.

In July 2006, Felipe Calderón, also from the PAN, won the presidential elections by a margin of 0.6 percent against candidate Andrés Manuel López Obrador from the Partido de la Revolución Democrática (PRD), then one of the three largest parties after the PRI and the PAN.[9] The elections were highly contested because two distinct views on how to govern Mexico were in competition. Calderón promised to continue market-driven policies and reforms, whereas López Obrador based his campaign on a direct criticism of "neoliberal" policies, arguing that they had triggered deep social inequalities. On 7 December 2006, just a few days after taking office, Calderón launched his 'fight against drugs'. Astorga (2011, 2016) has claimed that drug trafficking, and even the nexus between politicians and drug cartels, are not recent issues; they have been part of Mexican history at least from the early 1900s. However, as Astorga argues, Calderón's 'fight against drugs' took a completely different approach to manage this problem.

Although some have praised Calderón's 'fight on drugs' as "inevitable" (Chabat, 2010), other scholars have questioned the efficacy and pertinence of this 'war' (Correa-Cabrera, 2017; Mercille, 2011; Morton, 2012; Scheneck, 2012); a war that has had an unfortunately high toll of human lives (Frías & Finkelhor, 2018; González, 2009). As a Mexican national, I have experienced the war's atrocious consequences. Friends of mine have been disappeared and I have witnessed how peaceful cities and towns turned into ravaged places of armed confrontations. The human devastation of this 'war' in Veracruz, the state where I lived, worked and conducted this research, has been widely documented (Angel, 2017; Mundaca, 2014; Zavaleta, 2020). In 2017, for example, Mexico's largest clandestine grave was found a few dozen kilometers from the Emiliano Zapata and Benito Juárez primary schools.

After 12 years in opposition, in 2012 the PRI returned to power under Enrique Peña Nieto. Olvera (2016, p. 288) claims that the ultimate aim of the Peña Nieto administration (2012–2018) was to "accomplish the neoliberal cycle" started by fellow PRI members in the 1980s and continued by PAN governments from 2000 to 2012. Through deep reforms to energy, labor and education, Peña Nieto's government strengthened the aggressive expansion of private interests in public areas. Through the energy reform, after 80 years of exclusive state control, doors were opened for foreign companies to participate in drilling oil and gas reserves in Mexico. The labor reform introduced outsourcing and created better conditions for enterprises, to the detriment of workers' rights. The education reform culminated two decades of changes towards the modelling of education under market logics and the standardization of teaching.

These structural reforms were largely celebrated by some national and foreign commentators. For example, in the 24 February 2014 edition of *Time*, Peña Nieto was showcased as the "savior" of Mexico and his reforms were praised as "the most ambitious" reforms "in memory" (Crowley, 2014, para. 3). Nevertheless, not everyone has been that optimistic about those reforms. In September 2013, for example, a massive teachers' strike began in many states around the country after the Mexican Congress approved the 2013 Education Reform. The protests arose, at least in part, because the reform was conceived by Mexican teachers as an imposition from the Organisation for Economic Co-operation and Development (OECD) that sought to impose a managerial perspective on schools, teachers' work and the learning process itself. Overall, Peña Nieto's reforms were legislated and enacted amidst popular resistance and accusations of corruption (Flores-Macías, 2016; Gómez, 2014).

According to Transparency International (2018), Mexico scored 28 points out of 100 in the 2018 corruption index, ranking 138 in the list of 180 countries. Compared to other Latin American countries, with similar conditions like language, history of Spanish colonialism and difficult economic conditions, Mexico's place in the ranking is considerably low. Uruguay and Chile, for example, rank 23 (70/100 points) and 27 (67/100), respectively. Mexico has decreased 7 positions since 2013, which coincides with the Peña-Nieto administration. For Transparency International (n.d.), political corruption occurs when "policies, institutions and rules of procedure" are manipulated "in the allocation of resources and financing by political decision makers". I offer multiple examples of political corruption and its effects over the promotion of healthy lifestyles in schools through this book.

Schools, Nutrition and Public Health: Constructing a Modern Population

I have painted a broad picture of how the Mexican state has been politically and economically constructed and how it has changed between the early 1900s and today. In this and the following sections, I offer a more localized description about the central place of policy in the making of 'modern' Mexico over the twentieth century, specifically in education and health practices. In this section, I describe how policymakers used education and nutrition policy to construct a 'modern' population and to enlarge the corporatist Mexican state. In the next section, I show how public health policy in Mexico has been partially influenced by U.S. interests and shaped by market enthusiasts. From a theoretical point of view, this section provides the contexts where healthy lifestyles started to be constructed as a *dispositif.*

In the last two decades of the nineteenth century, under Porfirio Díaz's dictatorship, foreign companies had invested heavily in the oil, railroad and mining industries (Joseph & Buchenau, 2013). The arrival of new forms of production required the establishment of a trained and "obedient" workforce, and the dissipation of "local knowledge" to "replace it with new, abstract notions of time and space" (Buffington & French, 2000, pp. 421–422). This echoed the Porfirian political elite's dream of crafting a 'modern' Mexico.[10] Before the revolution took shape, a group of Porfirian intellectuals and self-proclaimed positivists known as *los científicos* (the scientists),[11] had embarked on turning Mexico's traditional and rural society, and its indigenous peoples, into 'modern' Mexican citizens (Raat, 1971). The científicos related the country's underdevelopment to the lack of education (Lewis, 2006) and the corn-based diet (Pío Martínez, 2013).

For example, Francisco Bulnes (1899), an educated and well-travelled científico, attributed the "backwardness" of poor and rural Mexicans to their corn-based diet and other pre-Hispanic and colonial cultural manifestations. Although an educated population had been deemed an important component in modernizing Mexico, during the Díaz administration education was mainly at the service of the middle-class: a national education system did not exist. Instead, municipalities and the Catholic Church managed schools and delivered curriculum. The few existing schools in the country were poorly resourced and located in shabby tenements. By the end of the nineteenth century, schools were federalized and hygiene became a key issue in the process of modernization and the creation of a national Mexican identity (Schell, 2004).

In the first years of the twentieth century, education was prioritized by both pre- and post-revolutionary leaders. Funds allocated for educational purposes increased, the number of enrolled students doubled and teachers' education was institutionalized (Buffington & French, 2000). In 1905, the Secretaría de Educación Pública (SEP) was created and put into the hands of Justo Sierra, a científico. During the intense years of armed conflict between 1910 and 1920, actions to expand education were on hold. In 1921, President Álvaro Obregón appointed José Vasconcelos as the head of the recently restructured SEP. Vasconcelos was a controversial intellectual who, before his appointment as the secretary of education, had been continuously travelling between Mexico, the USA and other Latin American and European countries (Stavans, 2011). Between 1922 and 1923, Vasconcelos deployed *Misiones Culturales* (Cultural Missions) and a rural education program to build a national Mexican identity, drawing on his own contentious perspective on race, indigenous people, nation building, which were ideas from the científicos (Beezley, 2011). Through these programs, teachers and "cultural missionaries" were sent to remote and indigenous areas across the country to instruct the population in reading and writing but also to forge a 'modern' Mexican culture through art, culture, music, hygiene and nutrition campaigns.

In the project of 'modernizing' Mexico, the transformation of the population's nutrition and hygiene practices were important goals for policymakers. Schools represented the ideal spaces to realize these goals. In this sense, Bliss (2006, p. 205) argues that given the state's limited penetration in Mexican homes, "hygiene education emerged as a way for the state to challenge 'unhealthy' private behaviors". According to Pilcher (1998, p. 92), education programs in post-revolutionary Mexico also "provided more direct means of inculcating middle-class dietary goals in the countryside". Pilcher describes how teachers working in rural areas disseminated the idea that their corn-based diet represented social backwardness and encouraged peasants to change their diet for wheat-made foods, seen as a sign of cultural and economic progress.

The institutionalization of public education and the deployment of educational programs were successful in increasing the number of literate Mexicans and made a free, secular education accessible to almost everyone. By the mid-1920s, there were about 2000 federal-run schools in Mexico. By 1936, the number of schools had increased to approximately 11,000 with about 14,000 teachers (Benjamin, 2000). According to census records, in the 1920s about 70 percent of Mexicans were illiterate, but this percentage had been considerably reduced by the beginning of 1940 (Dirección General de Estadística, 1943). However, the attempted cultural changes pursued by education and nutrition policies, like making children prefer bread over tortillas, did not always translate easily in schools and communities (Pilcher, 1998; Vaughan, 2006). In many cases, as Vaughan (1997, 2006) has documented, teachers had to negotiate with community leaders to introduce the ideas that policymakers had devised to 'modernize' rural lifestyles through schooling.

Mexicans resisted the cultural impositions deployed through post-revolutionary education programs in many ways. Nonetheless, from the 1920s to the 1940s, as these programs were implemented, the presence of the nascent corporatist Mexican state, and the political power of the "party of the revolution", as the PRI became to be widely known, were spread throughout Mexico. From the Obregón to the Cárdenas governments, education programs served to tackle the country's alleged backwardness, but also enlarged the state's and the party's power. In the 1930s, schooling was used to reaffirm the emerging political power of the "party of the revolution" through the active engagement of teachers in organizing the workers' associations that would give birth to corporatist Mexico. The conciliatory role that teachers played between federal policy and local interests resulted in the politicization of the teaching profession and the teachers' union. It was for this reason that some teachers in Mexico became a source of political control during elections (Vaughan, 2006). A legacy that, as I mentioned earlier in this chapter and as I will describe in Chapter 5, remains part of Mexican education today.

Public Health Policy, U.S. Influence and the Emergence of Healthy Lifestyles

When Venustiano Carranza announced the new Mexican Constitution of 1917, Mexico–U.S. diplomatic relations became tense because Article 27 and Article 123 threatened the interests of U.S. oil companies based in Mexico (Hall, 1995). According to historians, Mexico–U.S. relations improved in 1920 when Álvaro Obregón became president (Buchenau, 2011; Garrido, 1991; Hart, 1997). Obregón needed U.S. recognition and support to fight the conflicts that continued across the country and to consolidate his government. To show his willingness to improve relations between the two countries, Obregón agreed that Mexico would participate in the Rockefeller Foundation's yellow fever and hookworm campaigns (Birn, 1996, 2003; Birn & Solórzano, 1999; Solórzano, 1992). In the early 1920s, the main issues affecting the health of Mexicans were gastrointestinal diseases, malaria and tuberculosis. However, according to Solórzano (1992), the Rockefeller Foundation directors were interested in a yellow fever campaign because it represented a convenient vehicle to influence public health policy and to expand U.S. interests in Mexico.

The Rockefeller Foundation yellow fever campaign involved exhaustive "house visiting, constant identification with the people, and the sharing of their customs and food habits, and above all it involved an explanation that whatever the Rockefeller personnel did, they did in the name of Mexico and its people" (Solórzano, 1992, p. 546). This campaign had concluded by the mid-1920s, but U.S. economic, political and cultural interests were further expanded across Mexico through another Rockefeller Foundation public health campaign. This time the health issue to be 'fought' was hookworm. Similar to what had happened earlier, the decision to launch a hookworm campaign was related to politics rather than to public health.

Birn (2003) shows that issues like malaria, diarrhoea and tuberculosis were more-pressing issues that required intervention in Mexico, however hookworm became the new Rockefeller Foundation target because it served the Foundation's political and economic interests. While these campaigns brought some public health improvements for the Mexican population (Birn, 1996, 2003; Birn & Solórzano, 1999), historians have shown that the Rockefeller Foundation's public health campaigns were directed at strategic locations with large investment from oil corporations from the United States. From the early 1900s, as Santiago (2006) has thoroughly documented, U.S.-based firms started to develop the oil industry across northern Veracruz, which by the 1920s made Mexico the third largest oil producers in the world. Nevertheless, as the "first site of oil production in the tropical areas of the world", U.S. oil corporations faced the challenge of controlling the "whole gamut of diseases that thrived in those environmental and social conditions" (Santiago, 2006, pp. 2–6). It is therefore unsurprising why the Rockefeller Foundation was so invested in 'fighting' hookworm and malaria in Veracruz. Thus, through their public health campaigns, the Rockefeller Foundation facilitated the expansion of U.S. capitalism and shaped the Mexican public health system.

Education was a vital component in modelling public health in Mexico under the U.S. public health rationality. According to Birn (1996), from the 1920s to the 1950s, dozens of Mexican health officials and researchers received grants to be trained in U.S. health institutions. One of these officials was Guillermo Soberón, who obtained a PhD from the University of Wisconsin in the mid-1950s (Wences, 2018). After completing his PhD, Soberón established a new biochemistry research center and reformulated the medicine program at the prestigious Universidad Nacional Autónoma de México (UNAM). Through these actions, Soberón was training future health researchers and administrators and developing a vast network within the health sector. Apart from his academic talent, Soberón showed political skill that escalated him up the UNAM hierarchy, becoming chancellor between 1973 and 1981.

De la Madrid appointed Soberón as the Mexican secretary of health at the end of his term in the UNAM chancellery. As secretary of health (1982–1988), Soberón initiated a series of transformations in the public health sector, aiming to install a pro-market model of health care in Mexico. For this purpose, Soberón partnered with powerful businessmen from the pharmaceutical, banking, food and retailing sectors to establish FUNSALUD (see Chapter 1). To secure the expansion of the pro-market model within the health system, as Abrantes Pêgo (2010) has meticulously documented, Soberón created and consolidated a group of officials and researchers. Although Mexico was experiencing a deep economic crisis, Soberón lobbied to obtain public and private funds to create the current Instituto Nacional de Salud Pública (INSP) and to support the education of his team members. Thus, the training of Mexican public health officials and researchers in U.S. universities intensified through the 1980s. I term the members of Soberón's group "health technocrats" because of the similarities between them and the PRI technocrats described above.

Nonetheless, the reforms the group were planning for Mexico's health system met with resistance from different sectors. The health technocrats therefore launched a reorientation of the public health paradigm in Mexico: they gradually introduced market logic to the health system, and the neoliberal rationalities of choice and self-responsibility to govern the population's health. For this purpose, Julio Frenk, a scholar trained at the University of Michigan, incorporated the tenets of "the new public health" to research and organize public health in Mexico in the late 1980s/early 1990s. This laid the theoretical groundwork for how health should be conceived, researched, treated and governed in Mexico (see Frenk, 1988, 1993; Frenk et al., 1991). Thus, new concepts, analytical dimensions, academic publishing dynamics, funding mechanisms and forms of administration were introduced through the work of Frenk and other health technocrats (Abrantes Pêgo, 2010).

In line with the new public health, the issues affecting Mexican's health towards the end of the twentieth century were associated with, or constructed as an intrinsic result of, technological development, economic growth and a linear perspective of progress. Therefore, parallel to broader market-based reforms in the health sector, public health interventions aimed at minimizing "risk" and regulating "lifestyle" were launched to address the negative effects on health introduced by the process of modernization (Frenk et al., 1991). Obesity, as I will show in Chapter 3, has been constructed in Mexico as one of the intrinsic and inevitable outcomes of "development". The solutions, therefore, have been developed with the aim of providing the population with the required information to make "good choices" and maintain a "healthy lifestyle". Schools have served a key function in this task, given their capacity to reach a large segment of the Mexican population. Lifestyle change is at the core of the *Lineamientos*, the policy that regulates school food in Mexico.

School Food: From Collective Organization to Individual Care

A cooperativa escolar [school cooperative] is the name given to the space where multiple practices and transactions around food occur in Mexican schools. It is neither a tuck-shop nor a canteen, in the sense these terms are used in English-speaking countries. Cooperativas escolares in Mexico, as I will describe at length in Chapter 5, can comprise more than one physical space: a kitchen within the school; a table set up to sell diverse products during the break; and the principal's office, as was the case at Emiliano Zapata Primary School. What is cooked, sold and eaten in the cooperativas escolares, as I sketched out in Chapter 1, is influenced by the local economy and culture, but it is also shaped by policy.

Food in schools started to be regulated in the mid-1930s, when the Mexican government released the *Reglamento 1934*. The main purpose of this policy was to set out rules for the cooperative organization of the consumption of different products, food among them, within schools. From their inception, cooperativas escolares were conceived as organizations managed by teachers and students to generate revenue for the school from the sale of products. If the *Reglamento 1934* is situated in the political and economic context that I described earlier, we can see that the creation of cooperativas escolares was aligned with the government project of a nascent corporatist state in Mexico, which required mobilizing people to strengthen its political bases. This point was made clear in the *Reglamento 1934* (p. 598), where PRI policymakers stated that members of the cooperativas escolares had to "promote the formation of a Federation of School Cooperatives"; a demand connected to the PRI's intention to bring together workers, peasants, teachers and the community towards the achievement of its own goals of government.

The Cárdenas administration amended the *Reglamento 1934*, and the updated *Reglamento 1937* (p. 1) criticized the previous policy because it was not aligned with Mexico's development project and because it promoted a "consumerist" logic without using "production" to promote "educative knowledge". Therefore, the *Reglamento 1937* assigned a "pedagogical dimension" to the production, sale and consumption of school food. This policy described how cooperativas escolares should be managed. Article 19 specified that the assets of cooperativas escolares should be divided into five "funds". The "reserve fund", comprised of 10 percent of revenues, would be the cooperativa escolar's "collective property" and its economic resources. The "social provision fund" (10 percent) could be used to support members involved in accidents or illness, while the "leisure fund" (10 percent) was designed to promote social and cultural activities in the community. The "development fund" (10 percent) was aimed at boosting the cooperativa escolar's operations, and finally, the "distributable fund" (60 percent) would be distributed to the members of the cooperativa escolar at the end of the school year (pp. 1–3).

The regulation of school food in the 1930s was connected to the broader project of government that was underway in those years. Schools and teachers linked rural communities with the ongoing processes of state formation and modernization, vehicles through which the state could reach the intimate private lives of families. The cooperativas escolares were envisaged as pedagogical tools to teach the production and sale of different products inside and outside of schools and, thus, were used to mobilize teachers and students to contribute to the industrial and capitalist development of Mexico. Therefore, the *Reglamento* of 1934 and 1937 not only regulated school food but, as Civera Cerecedo (2010) has noted, they also organized the school community to assist in the government project.

The *Reglamento 1934* and the *Reglamento 1937* presented, in paper, an ideal form of organizing the production and sale of food in schools. According to this perspective, school actors would work cooperatively to generate an income to be later re-distributed and used to aid operations in schools. Yet in reality this ideal did not translate perfectly. Historical work on education in early twentieth century in Mexico offers multiple examples of tensions in the implementation of these policies. Montes de Oca Navas (2013) and Civera Cerecedo (2010), for example, describe the difficulties of setting up and running a cooperativa escolar, the struggles to control the cooperativa and its income, and the misuse of the economic resources resulting from the transactions of food in schools in the 1930s.[12] In these years, cooperativas escolares did more than produce and sell food. They were a vehicle for organization and a pedagogical framework to teach students through experience and production, particularly in the agricultural space.

The *Reglamento 1937* remained unchanged for 25 years. Yet, the rapid industrialization and urbanization experienced during the "Mexican Miracle" (1940–1960), together with the changing political landscape required changes to this policy. Complaints against cooperativas escolares now started to be made not only based on the misuses of income but also on health grounds.[13] In 1962, the *Reglamento 1937* was superceded by the *Reglamento 1962*. In this new policy, the cooperativas escolares were officially freed from their role as political organizer and were situated as having "an exclusively educative purpose" (p. 3).

The *Reglamento* was again modified in 1982, with one of the most interesting amendments endowing cooperativas escolares with a new responsibility: they had to contribute funds to "improve the school facilities and equipment" and for "the development of teaching activities in general" (*Reglamento 1982*, p. 21). Due to the economic crisis of the 1980s, as discussed previously, education expenditure had been reduced. Consequently, schools received less funds, equipment and resources (Vázquez, 1997). With reduced funding and more responsibilities, schools started to self-fund many activities. Revenue from food sales became an essential source of funding for schools, as the reader will come to appreciate in Chapter 5.

The *Reglamento 1982* remained the policy framing the production and sales of food within Mexican schools until 2010, when the *Lineamientos 2010* replaced it. After almost 80 years, the focus of the regulation changed substantially. It went from organizing food sales within schools for the benefit of the institution—at least in theory, to measuring the number of calories, nutrients and portions that students should consume within school hours. The *Lineamientos*, in 2010 and in the 2014 update, eliminated cooperativas escolares. Instead, the new policy called for a decentralization of the production and sale of food within schools and opened space for "providers" who must meet nutritional, hygienic and administrative requirements in order to supply food. The *Lineamientos* also introduced a new language to talk about food and the forms in which it should be prepared, sold and consumed in Mexican schools. Unlike all versions of the *Reglamento*, where school food was deemed a vehicle for collective organizing,[14] food in the *Lineamientos* was depicted as a tool to pursue health. Therefore, food was categorized as "healthy/unhealthy", and a complex array of discursive elements and practices were put into play around it.

Policies are inserted in and constitute part of a larger arrangement of politics, culture and the economy. The language of policy is contextual. It is partly made up from broader political and economic issues. Also, policies have a temporality, but they do not simply cease to exist. On paper, every new version of the *Reglamento* eroded the previous one; as the *Lineamientos 2010* officially buried the *Reglamento 1982*. Yet in reality these vestiges of "old" policies coexist with the new in governing the practices around food in schools. In some instances, the school community remains unaware of the policy change, yet at other times they incorporate elements of the new policy into their repertoire of practices framed by a previous one. For instance, while the *Lineamientos* 2010 and 2014 technically eliminated the cooperativas escolares, this name is still widely used by people to refer to the spaces where food is produced, sold and consumed in schools. This was also the case during my fieldwork.

In mid-June 2016, I talked to Isela—the person in charge of overseeing the "cooperativas escolares" across the Veracruz Metropolitan School District—about school food regulations, her perspectives on the relationship between school food and health, and her role in and experiences with implementing school food policies. Isela joined this position in the district in 2007 after 20 years in teaching and leadership roles in schools. She had extensive, both theoretical and practical, knowledge of food regulations. Isela participated in the implementation of the *Lineamientos 2010* in her district. She told me how hard it had been to "convince" schools to stop selling highly profitable ultra-processed products and other 'unhealthy' foods—mainly *masa*-based foods. Opposition was large, but schools ended up adopting some of the requirements of the *Lineamientos 2010*. They, for instance, decreased the offer of carbonated-sugary drinks [*refrescos*] (see Chapter 6). However, this adoption of a new practice occurred in conjunction with the recommendations and organization given by the *Reglamento 1982*.

Isela was an advocate of the *Lineamientos 2010* and the 2014 update and worked hard to put them to work. She was nonetheless also aware of the limitations in schools and the central role food sales have in their operations. Isela showed me a notebook where she compiles all the information from the 80 cooperativas escolares across the Veracruz Metropolitan School District. Regardless of the policy change, Isela, like all the people I spoke with during my fieldwork, always use the term cooperativas escolares when talking about food provisioning in schools. She had the "official list" of products sold, but she also knew that other products were commonly sold in schools. Each school provides a small percentage of their revenue from the sale of food to the district. She also knew about disputes concerning food sales and the misuse of money in schools. However, in spite of some negative issues, Isela considered that, overall, schools did a good job in feeding children under mostly pressing circumstances.

Benito Juárez Primary School was, according to Isela and also from some of my own experiences, one of the schools where the provision of food was very complex. A few days before my interview with Isela, a representative of the Parents Committee had stolen the net income of one year from Nutrilandia. The school was embroiled in a chaotic scandal. In a public meeting with authorities from the school and the district, parents complained about the high prices of the ultra-processed products offered in the school and questioned how the profits were used. However, parents did not question *why* ultra-processed products were sold inside the school. The scandal occurred at a very interesting moment: elections. As the re-direction of government funding towards the school enabled the construction of a new dining area to "attract" votes, the scandal in the management of food was damaging the image of both the school and the government.

The *Lineamientos* eliminated the cooperativas escolares. This policy enabled external actors to prepare, sell and profit from in-school food. However, in 2016 schools were still framing their practices around food after the *Reglamento 1982*, and following only a few of the recommendations in the *Lineamientos*. At the end of my conversation with Isela, she gave me photocopies of the *Reglamento 1982* and said that that document was what "guided" the regulation of food in schools. Similarly, most of the education authorities and school actors that I talked to always spoke about school food in connection with the cooperativas escolares.

Although the imperative for governing food in schools in the name of health may be relatively new, the regulation of food production and sale in these spaces has taken other forms in the past. Healthy lifestyles, as a tool of government, has emerged under particular circumstances: it was made possible not only by a change in economic policy, but also by the development of new scientific approaches to the theorization and research of public health and in the making of public health policy. These new approaches are framed by the dynamics of a market-driven economy, which, as Chapter 3 will show, is evident in the language used in policy.

Conclusion

In this chapter I have described, from a historical perspective, three fundamental points for the theoretical and empirical elaboration of this book. First, I explained how the Mexican state emerged, parallel to the formation of the PRI as the "party of the revolution", through the first half of the twentieth century amidst power struggles of local and international actors. I emphasized the transformations that the PRI went through in its 70 years of government, especially in the 1980s, to show how local conditions facilitated the adoption of neoliberalism as the political and economic model in Mexico. This description offers the groundwork for the theoretical discussion about neoliberalism and policy that follows in Chapter 3. It is worth highlighting that, although it has been adopted globally, neoliberalism has not been practiced equally in all countries around the world. Therefore, the first section of this chapter provided an overview of how local political and economic conditions shaped the adoption of neoliberalism in Mexico.

Second, I offered a localized description about the place of policy in the making of 'modern' Mexico in the twentieth century. For this purpose, I described how Mexican policymakers used education and nutrition policy to construct a 'modern' population and to enlarge the corporatist state. Furthermore, I showed that health policy in Mexico has been influenced, to some extent, by U.S. interests and, since the 1980s, shaped by a group of "technocrats" managing the health sector. I will further elaborate this point in Chapter 3 to show how, within the *dispositif of healthy lifestyles*, the voices of these pro-market actors have been very influential in shaping obesity policy.

Third, this brief narrative of twentieth-century Mexico has shown the complex politics that have historically taken place in and around Mexican schools. Through the case of school food regulation, I revealed how schools' responsibilities change according to specific political contexts. As in the past, schools are central in government projects today. This is one reason why corporations have become so invested in entering schools and using them as platforms to disseminate their perspectives on 'health' and 'ideal' forms of living.

Notes

1 Framing a critique on how the idea of modernity has driven the making of policy, and state formation in itself, is beyond the scope of this book. However, my understanding of modernity is influenced by my reading of decolonial and postdevelopment critiques of this idea, mainly by Latin American scholars who have discussed how a Euro-centrist, Western view has arbitrarily constructed peoples from non-European countries as less developed (see Escobar, 2011; Lander, 2003; Mignolo, 2011).

2 Plutarco Elías are the general's first name and middle name; Calles is his surname. From here on, I refer to him by his surname.

3 I am not offering a full historical analysis of Mexican politics in the early twentieth century here. Instead, I am engaging in this brief discussion to provide the reader with a brief context of how the PRI, and a modern state, were created in Mexico, and, in later sections, the connections between this process and the regulation of food in schools. Also, it is important to note that the first section of this chapter describes a mostly "internal" process of state construction, without much attention given to how "external" factors contributed to the formation of Mexico and the PRI throughout the twentieth century. One such external factor, for instance, is the constant inference of the United States in Mexican politics and policy (see Hall, 1995, for an example of this during the 1920s). Many of the events that took place in Mexico in the first decades of the twentieth century—and more broadly what happens in the country today—cannot

be explained without tracing connections to dynamics generated in, or fostered by groups from, the Unit States. During the Porfirio Díaz government, for example, U.S.-owned railroad, mining and oil corporations were granted generous concessions of lands and the right to extract resources. These specials concessions were cancelled by provisional revolutionary governments after 1910, which outraged U.S. corporations and government (Hall, 1995).

4   Mexicans have two last names. Here, "Ávila Camacho" comprises the president's surname. In this book, I refer to politicians using their two last names when this is the common practice. At other times, I only use one last name, as I have done with Calles and Cárdenas.

5   Original emphasis. González Casanova's (1986) book is in Spanish. My translation has slightly changed the original sense in the phrase: "un nuevo *estilo del Estado*".

6   I use this term in two, perhaps contradictory, ways. First, by Third World I refer to countries that have been subject to imperial colonialism or an institutionalised neo-colonialism by, mostly, European countries and the United States. In a less narrow view, following Gupta (2012, p. 303), I also use Third World to refer "to the effects of hegemonic representations of the West" and to "a particular historical conjuncture of place, power and knowledge". I situate Mexico, and myself, as part of the Third World. For a seminal critique of the construction of the Third World, see Escobar (2011).

7   Lewis' (1959, 1961) ethnographies of families living in popular suburbs in Mexico City in the 1940s and 1950s describe a different side of the story. In *Five Families: Mexican Case Studies in the Culture of Poverty*, Lewis (1959, p. 9) reported that, "over 60 per cent of the population were still ill-fed, ill-housed, and ill-clothed in 1956, 40 per cent were illiterate, and 46 per cent of the nation's children were not going to school". Lewis also highlighted the increasing dependency that the Mexican economy started to have on the United States: "[f]rom 1942 to 1955 about a million and a half Mexicans came to the United States", and "[i]n 1957 over 700,000 tourists from the United States spent almost 600 million dollars in Mexico", an income "about equal to the total Mexican federal budget". In terms of housing, a central theme in his ethnographies, Lewis stated that according to the Mexican census of 1950 (see Dirección General de Estadística, 1955), "60 per cent" of the dwellings in the country "had only one room and 25 per cent two rooms", "70 per cent of all houses were made of adobe [clay], wood, poles and rods, or rubble" and "[o]nly 17 per cent had private, piped water" (p. 10). Lewis' work was hugely polemic among government officials and intellectuals in Mexico in the 1960s, mainly because Lewis represented an image of Mexico contradicting the official narrative, which according to some, validating the U.S. expansionist agenda (see Pozas, 1961).

8   Camp argues that the term "political technocrats" is more appropriate in the Mexican context, because there is no clear line of distinction between a "technocrat" and a "politician". I use technocrats for space and fluency.

9   Prior to the elections, López Obrador had been the frontrunner. Two months before election day, a fierce mass media campaign attacking López Obrador and his political project was launched. According to political scientists (Greene, 2011; Klesner, 2007; Moreno, 2007; Sánchez Murillo & Aceves González, 2010), the stigmatization campaign successfully created fear of López Obrador's presidency.

10 I use "Porfirian political elite" to refer to the politicians who were influential during the Porfirio Díaz dictatorship.

11 For an overview of the origins, political careers and ideological influences of *los científicos*, see Priego (2016).

12 In these years, the cooperativas escolares comprised more activities than food sales, see Civera Cerecedo (2010) and Montes de Oca Nava (2013).

13 In September 1963, the conservative newspaper, *El Informador* (1963), which repeatedly criticised the cooperativas escolares, argued that these spaces had turned into a "real plague for the health of students". The article claims that hand-made foods are

dangerous and therefore only "strictly sanitarily regulated products" should be sold in schools.

14 I have told a rather romantic story about cooperativas escolares. However, from personal experience I also know that they are deeply complex and problematic. Historically, the purpose and management of the cooperativas escolares have also been subject to criticism (see *El Informador*, 1963; Gerardo Rodríguez, 2010; Montes de Oca Navas, 2013).

References

Abrantes Pêgo, R. (2010). *Salubristas y neosalubristas en la reforma del Estado: Grupos de interés en México e instituciones públicas de salud, 1982–2000* [*The rise of the new public health: Neoliberal reforms and stakeholders in Mexico, 1982–2000*]. El Colegio de Michoacán.

Angel, A. (2017). Otra fosa clandestina de Veracruz: 10 mil fragmentos humanos en un rancho y sólo 4 identificados [Discovering a new clandestine grave in rural Veracruz: 10 thousand bones, 4 identified corpses]. *Animal Político*. https://www.animalpolitico.com/2017/04/fosa-clandestina-en-rancho-veracruz/.

Astorga, L. (2011). *Qué querían que hiciera? Inseguridad y delicuencia organizada en el gobierno de Felipe Calderón* [*What did you want me to do: Insecurity and organised crime under Felipe Calderón's government*]. Grijalbo.

Astorga, L. (2016). *El siglo de las drogas: Del Porfiriato al nuevo milenio* [*The century of drugs: From the Porfiriato to the new millennium*]. Debolsillo.

Babb, S. L. (2001). *Managing Mexico: Economists from nationalism to neoliberalism*. Princeton University Press.

Baer, M. D. (2004). Mexico at an impasse. *Foreign Affairs*, 83(1), 101–113.

Ballinas, V., & Méndez, E. (2006). Fox triplicó las concesiones del líquido; Coca-Cola y Nestlé, las beneficiadas: PRD [Fox tripled water concessions to benefit Coca-Cola and Nestlé: PRD]. *La Jornada*. https://www.jornada.com.mx/2006/03/17/index.php?section=sociedad&article=050n1soc.

Beezley, W. H. (2011). Creating a revolutionary culture: Vasconcelos, Indians, anthropologists, and calendar girls. In W. H. Beezley (ed.), *A companion to Mexican history and culture* (pp. 420–438). Blackwell Publishing.

Benjamin, T. (2000). Rebuilding the nation. In M. C. Meyer & W. H. Beezley (eds.), *The Oxford history of Mexico* (pp. 467–502). Oxford University Press.

Birn, A.-E. (1996). Public health or public menace? The Rockefeller Foundation and public health in Mexico, 1920–1950. *Voluntas: International Journal of Voluntary and Nonprofit Organizations*, 7(1), 35–56. http://doi.org/10.1007/bf02354067.

Birn, A.-E. (2003). Revolution, the scatological way: The Rockefeller Foundation's hookworm campaign in 1920s Mexico. In D. Armus (ed.), *Disease in the history of modern Latin America: From malaria to AIDS* (pp. 158–182). Duke University Press.

Birn, A.-E., & Solórzano, A. (1999). Public health policy paradoxes: Science and politics in the Rockefeller Foundation's hookworm campaign in Mexico in the 1920s. *Social Science & Medicine*, 49(9), 1197–1213. https://doi.org/10.1016/S0277-9536(99)00160-00164.

Bliss, K. E. (2006). For the health of the nation: Gender and the cultural politics of social hygiene in Revolutionary Mexico. In M. K. Vaughan & S. E. Lewis (eds.), *The eagle and the virgin: Nation and cultural revolution in Mexico, 1920–1940* (pp. 196–218). Duke University Press.

Buchenau, J. (2006). *Plutarco Elías Calles and the Mexican Revolution*. Rowman & Littlefield Publishers.

Buchenau, J. (2011). *The last caudillo: Alvaro Obregón and the Mexican Revolution*. Wiley-Blackwell.

Buffington, R. M., & French, W. E. (2000). The culture of modernity. In M. C. Meyer & W. H. Beezley (eds.), *The Oxford history of Mexico* (pp. 397–434). Oxford University Press.

Bulnes, F. (1899). *El porvernir de las naciones Hispano Americanas ante las conquistas recientes de Europa y los Estados Unidos* [*The future of nations in the face of the recent invasions from Europe and the United States*]. Imprenta de Mariano Nava.

Bunker, S. B., & Macías-González, V. M. (2011). Consumption and material culture in Twentieth Century. In W. H. Beezley (ed.), *A companion to Mexican history and culture* (pp. 83–118). Blackwell Publishing.

Caldera Ortega, A. R. (2017). Cambio y confrontación de proyectos políticos en la gestión del agua en México [Change, struggles and politics of water management in Mexico]. In C. Denzin, F. Taboada, & R. Pacheco Vega (eds.), *El agua en México: Actores, sectores y paradigmas para una transformación social-ecológica* [*Water in Mexico: Actors, sectors and paradigms for a socio-ecological transformation*] (pp. 215–248). Friedrich-Ebert-Stiftung.

Camp, R. A. (1985). The political technocrat in Mexico and the survival of the political system. *Latin American Research Review*, 20(1), 97–118.

Camp, R. A. (2008). Political recruitment, governance, and leadership in Mexico: How democracy has made a difference. In P. M. Siavelis & S. Morgenstern (eds.), *Pathways to power: Political recruitment and candidate selection in Latin America* (pp. 292–315). The Pennsylvania State University Press.

Camp, R. A. (2011). The revolution's second generation: The miracle, 1946–1982 and collapse of the PRI 1982–2000. In W. H. Beezley (ed.), *A companion to Mexican history and culture* (pp. 468–479). Blackwell Publishing.

Carmona, F., Montaño, G., Carrión, J., & Aguilar, A. (1970). *El Milagro Mexicano* [*The Mexican miracle*]. Editorial Nuestro Tiempo.

Centeno, M. A., & Maxfield, S. (1992). The marriage of finance and order: Changes in the Mexican political elite. *Journal of Latin American Studies*, 24(1), 57–85. https://doi.org/10.1017/S0022216X00022951.

Chabat, J. (2010). *Combatting drugs in Mexico under Calderón: The inevitable war*, no. 205. Centro de Investigación y Docencia Económica. http://repositorio-digital.cide.edu/bitstream/handle/11651/826/103252.pdf?sequence=1&isAllowed=y.

Civera Cerecedo, A. (2010). El Cooperativismo en la Escuela Rural del México de los Años Treinta [Cooperativism in rural education in 1930s Mexico]. *Anuario de Estudios Americanos*, 67(2), 467–491.

Correa-Cabrera, G. (2017). *Los Zetas Inc.: Criminal corporations, energy, and civil war in Mexico*. University of Texas Press.

Crowley, M. (2014). The Committee to Save Mexico. *Time*. https://time.com/7058/the-committee-to-save-mexico/.

Delgado-Ramos, G. C. (2014). *Apropiación de agua, medio ambiente y obesidad: Los impactos del negocio de bebidas embotelladas en México* [*Water appropriation, the environment and obesity: The impact of bottled drinks in Mexico*]. Universidad Nacional Autónoma de México.

Dirección General de Estadística. (1943). *Sexto Censo de Población 1940. Estados Unidos Mexicanos* [*Sixth population census 1940. Mexico*]. Secretaría de la Economía Nacional, Dirección General de Estadística.

Dirección General de Estadística. (1955). *Séptimo Censo General de Población 1950. Estados Unidos Mexicanos* [*Seventh population census 1950. Mexico*]. Secretaría de la Economía Nacional, Dirección General de Estadística.

El Informador (1963, September 20). Cooperativas escolares [School cooperatives]. *El Informador.* http://www.hndm.unam.mx/consulta/publicacion/visualizar/558a37ea7d1ed64f16e027ff?intPagina=3&tipo=pagina&anio=1963&mes=09&dia=20.

Escobar, A. (2011). *Encountering development: The making and unmaking of the third world* (2nd ed.). Princeton University Press.

Flores-Macías, G. A. (2016). Latin America's new turbulence: Mexico's stalled reforms. *Journal of Democracy*, 27(2), 66–78. https://doi.org/10.1353/jod.2016.0022.

Ford, E. M. (2008). *Children of the Mexican miracle: Childhood and modernity in Mexico City, 1940–1968* [PhD, University of Illinois at Urbana-Champaign, Urbana, Illinois].

Fox, J. (1992). *The politics of food in Mexico: State power and social mobilization.* Cornell University Press.

Frenk, J. (1988). La salud pública: Campo del conocimiento y ámbito para la acción [Public health as field of knowledge and intervention]. *Salud Pública de México*, 30(2), 246–254.

Frenk, J., Bobadilla, J. L., Stern, C., Frejka, T., & Lozano, R. (1991). Elements for a theory of the health transition. *Health Transition Review*, 1(1), 21–38.

Frías, S. M., & Finkelhor, D. (2018). Homicide of children and adolescents in Mexico (1990–2013). *International Journal of Comparative and Applied Criminal Justice*, 42(4), 303–319. https://doi.org/10.1080/01924036.2017.1325760.

Garrido, L. J. (1991). *El Partido de la Revolución Institucionalizada. Medio siglo de poder político en México. La formación del nuevo estado (1928–1945)* [*The Party of the Institutionalised Revolution. 50 years of political power in Mexico. The formation of a new state (1928–1945)*]. Siglo XXI Editores.

Gerardo Rodríguez, P. (2010). La nueva fábula de las abejas. En torno a la regulación de los alimentos chatarra en las escuelas [The new fable of the bees. A discussion on the regulation of junk food in schools]. *Revista Latinoamericana de Estudios Educativos*, 40(3), 9–54.

Gochman, B. P. (1998). *Networks, neoliberalism, and NAFTA: Economic technocrats and policy change in Mexico, 1982–1997* [PhD, University of Denver, Denver].

Gómez, L. A. L. (2014). La desvalorización de la tierra en el patrón de producción, agudizada por las reformas energética y laboral de Enrique Peña Nieto (2012–2018) [The devaluation of land in the pattern of production, exacerbated by the energy and labor reforms of Enrique Peña Nieto (2012–2018)].*Estudios Socioterritoriales. Revista de Geografía*, 1(16), 47–80.

González, F. E. (2009). Mexico's drug wars get brutal. *Current History*, 108(715), 72–76.

Gónzalez Casanova, P. (1986). *El estado y los partidos políticos en México: Ensayos* [*The state and political parties in Mexico: Essays*]. Ediciones Era.

Greene, K. F. (2011). Campaign persuasion and nascent partisanship in Mexico's new democracy. *American Journal of Political Science*, 55(2), 398–416. https://doi.org/10.1111/j.1540-5907.2010.00497.x.

Gupta, A. (2012). *Red tape: Bureaucracy, structural violence, and poverty in India.* Duke University Press.

Hall, L. B. (1995). *Oil, banks, and politics: The United States and postrevolutionary Mexico, 1917–1924.* University of Texas Press.

Hart, J. M. (1997). *Revolutionary Mexico: The coming and process of the Mexican Revolution.* University of California Press.

Joseph, G. M., & Buchenau, J. (2013). *Mexico's once and future revolution: Social upheaval and the challenge of rule since the late nineteenth century.* Duke University Press.

Klesner, J. L. (2001). The end of Mexico's one-party regime. *PS: Political Science & Politics,* 34(1), 107–114. https://doi.org/10.1017/S1049096501000166.

Knight, A. (1985). The Mexican Revolution: Bourgeois? Nationalist? Or just a 'great rebellion'? *Bulletin of Latin American Research,* 4(2), 1–37.

Knight, A. (1996). Corruption in twentieth century Mexico. In W. Little & E. Posada-Carbó (eds.), *Political corruption in Europe and Latin America* (pp. 219–236). Macmillan Press.

Knight, A. (2010). The myth of the Mexican Revolution. *Past & Present,* No. 209, 223–273.

Lander, E. (ed.). (2003). *La colonialidad del saber: eurocentrismo y ciencias sociales [Coloniality of knowledge: Euro-centrism and social sciences].* CLACSO.

Larreguy, H., Montiel Olea, C. E., & Querubin, P. (2017). Political brokers: Partisans or agents? Evidence from the Mexican Teachers' Union. *American Journal of Political Science,* 61(4), 877–891. https://doi.org/10.1111/ajps.12322.

Laurell, A. C. (2015). Three decades of neoliberalism in Mexico: The destruction of society. *International Journal of Health Services,* 45(2), 246–264. https://doi.org/10.1177/0020731414568507.

Lewis, O. (1959). *Five families: Mexican case studies in the culture of poverty.* Basic Books.

Lewis, O. (1961). *The children of Sanchez: Autobiography of a Mexican family.* Random House.

Lewis, S. E. (2006). The nation, education, and the 'Indian problem' in Mexico, 1920–1940. In M. K. Vaughan & S. E. Lewis (eds.), *The eagle and the virgin: Nation and cultural revolution in Mexico, 1920–1940* (pp. 176–195). Duke University Press.

Lineamientos 2010 (Acuerdo mediante el cual se establecen los lineamientos generales para el expendio o distribución de alimentos y bebidas en los establecimientos de consumo escolar de los planteles de educación básica [General guidelines for the distribution or sales of food and drinks by retailers within basic education schools]) (2010). Diario Oficial de la Federación: Órgano del Gobierno Constitucional de los Estados Unidos Mexicanos.

Lineamientos 2014 (Acuerdo mediante el cual se establecen los lineamientos generales para el expendio y distribución de alimentos y bebidas preparados y procesados en las escuelas del Sistema Educativo Nacional [Guidelines for the sales and distribution of prepared and processed food and drinks in the Mexican national education system]) (2014). Diario Oficial de la Federación: Órgano del Gobierno Constitucional de los Estados Unidos Mexicanos.

Lomnitz, C. (2001). *Deep Mexico, silent Mexico: An anthropology of nationalism.* The University of Minnesota Press.

Mignolo, W. (2011). *The darker side of western modernity: Global futures, decolonial options.* Duke University Press.

Magaloni, B. (2008). *Voting for autocracy: Hegemonic party survival and its demise in Mexico.* Cambridge University Press.

Mercille, J. (2011). Violent narco-cartels or US hegemony? The political economy of the 'war on drugs' in Mexico. *Third World Quarterly,* 32(9), 1637–1653. https://doi.org/10.1080/01436597.2011.619881.

Montes de Oca Navas, E. (2013). Del discurso a la realidad: Los maestros Mexiquenses y la educación socialista (1934) [From discourse to reality: Teachers from the State of Mexico and the socialist education (1934)]. *La Colmena,* 80(October–December), 87–97.

Morales-Gómez, D. A., & Torres, C. A. (1990). *The state, corporatist politics, and educational policy making in Mexico*. Praeger Publishers.

Moreno, A. (2007). The 2006 Mexican presidential election: The economy, oil revenues, and ideology. *PS: Political Science & Politics*, 40(1), 15–19. https://doi.org/10.1017/S1049096507070035.

Morris, S. D. (1999). Corruption and the Mexican political system: Continuity and change. *Third World Quarterly*, 20(3), 623–643. https://doi.org/10.1080/01436599913721.

Morris, S. D. (2009). *Political corruption in Mexico: The impact of democratization*. Lynne Rienner Publishers.

Morton, A. D. (2012). The war on drugs in Mexico: A failed state? *Third World Quarterly*, 33(9), 1631–1645. https://doi.org/10.1080/01436597.2012.720837.

Mundaca, A. (2014). La Cuenca del Papaloapan se volvió territorio "zeta", y autoridades y ciudadanos lo sabían [The Papaloapan Basin turned into 'zeta-land', and people and authorities knew it]. *Sin Embargo*. https://www.sinembargo.mx/22-06-2014/1033465?utm_source=Correo.

Nash, J. (2007). Consuming interests: Water, rum, and Coca-Cola from ritual propitiation to corporate expropriation in highland Chiapas. *Cultural Anthropology*, 22(4), 621–639. https://doi.org/10.1525/can.2007.22.4.621.

Niblo, S. R. (1999). *Mexico in the 1940s: Modernity, politics, and corruption*. Rowman & Littlefield.

Ochoa, E. (2002). *Feeding Mexico: The political use of food since 1910*. Scholarly Resources Inc.

Olvera, A. J. (2016). La crisis política, los movimientos sociales y el futuro de la democracia en México [Political crisis, social movements and the future of democracy in Mexico]. *Revista Mexicana de Ciencias Políticas y Sociales*, 61(226), 279–296.

Otero, G. (1996). Neoliberal reform and politics in Mexico: An overview. In G. Otero (ed.), *Neoliberalism revisited: Economic restructuring and Mexico's political future* (pp. 1–25). Westview Press.

Pastor, R. (1993). NAFTA as the center of an integration process: The nontrade issues. *The Brookings Review*, 11(1), 40–45. https://doi.org/10.2307/20080364.

Pastor, M., & Wise, C. (1997). State policy, distribution and neoliberal reform in Mexico. *Journal of Latin American Studies*, 29(2), 419–456. https://doi.org/10.1017/S0022216X97004744.

Pastor, M., & Wise, C. (2005). The lost sexenio: Vicente Fox and the new politics of economic reform in Mexico. *Latin American Politics and Society*, 47(4), 135–160. https://doi.org/10.1111/j.1548-2456.2005.tb00331.x.

Pensado, J. M. (2013). *Rebel Mexico: Student unrest and authoritarian political culture during the long sixties*. Stanford University Press.

Pérez Monfort, R. (2011). On the street corner where stereotypes are born: Mexico City, 1940–1968. In W. H. Beezley (ed.), *A companion to Mexican history and culture* (pp. 34–53). Blackwell Publishing.

Pilcher, J. M. (1998). *Que vivan los tamales! Food and the making of Mexican identity*. University of New Mexico Press.

Pío Martínez, J. (2013). La ciencia de la nutrición y el control social en México en la primera mitad del Siglo XX [Nutrition science and social control during the first half of 20th-century Mexico]. *Relaciones*, 133(Winter), 225–255.

Pozas, R. (1961). La pobre antropología de Oscar Lewis [The poor anthropology of Oscar Lewis]. *Revista de la Universidad de México*, XVI(4), 12–13. https://www.revistadelauniversidad.mx/download/5a0bead1-206d-488c-a0c5-12d408b98a31?filename=4.

Priego, N. (2016). *Positivism, science and the 'scientists' in Porfirian Mexico: A reappraisal.* Liverpool University Press.

Raat, W. D. (1971). Los intelectuales, el positivismo y la cuestión indígena [Intellectuals, positivism and indigenism]. *Historia Mexicana*, 20(3), 412–427.

Reglamento 1934 (*Reglamento de las cooperativas escolares federales* [*Regulation of the federal school cooperatives*]). Diario Oficial de la Federación, Órgano del Gobierno Constitucional de los Estados Unidos Mexicanos, pp. 566–570.

Reglamento 1937 (*Reglamento de cooperativas escolares dependientes de la Secretaría de Educación Pública* [*Regulation of the school cooperatives from the Secretariat of Public Education*]). Diario Oficial de la Federación, Órgano del Gobierno Constitucional de los Estados Unidos Mexicanos, pp. 1–7.

Reglamento 1962 (*Reglamento de cooperativas escolares* [*Regulation of school cooperatives*]). Diario Oficial de la Federación, Órgano del Gobierno Constitucional de los Estados Unidos Mexicanos, pp. 3–6.

Reglamento 1982 (*Reglamento de cooperativas escolares* [*Regulation of school cooperatives*]). Diario Oficial de la Federación, Órgano del Gobierno Constitucional de los Estados Unidos Mexicanos, pp. 20–27.

Rubin, J. W. (1996). Decentering the regime: Culture and regional politics in Mexico. *Latin American Research Review*, 31(3), 85–126.

Ruíz, R. E. (1982). *The great rebellion: Mexico, 1905–1924.* W.W. Norton & Company.

Sánchez Murillo, L. F., & Aceves González, F. d. J. (2010). Campañas políticas y configuración del voto electoral en 2006. Encuestas electorales y publicidad política [Political campaigns and vote framing in 2006. Electoral surveys and political marketing]. *Revista Mexicana de Ciencias Políticas y Sociales* 50(202), 93–116.

Santiago, M. (2006). *The ecology of oil: Environment, labor, and the Mexican Revolution, 1900–1938.* Cambridge University Press.

Schell, P. A. (2004). Nationalizing children through schools and hygiene: Porfirian and revolutionary Mexico City. *The Americas*, 60(4), 559–587. https://doi.org/10.1353/tam.2004.0072.

Scheneck, G. D. (2012). A war on civilians: Disaster capitalism and the drug war in Mexico. *Seattle Journal for Social Justice*, 10(2), 927–980.

Schmitter, P. C. (1974). Still the century of corporatism? *The Review of Politics*, 36(1), 85–131.

Schryer, F. J. (2014). *They never come back: A story of undocumented workers from Mexico* (1st ed.). Cornell University Press.

Sherman, J. W. (2000). The Mexican 'Miracle' and its collapse. In M. C. Meyer & W. H. Beezley (eds.), *The Oxford history of Mexico* (pp. 575–607). Oxford University Press.

Smith, P. H. (2015). *Labyrinths of power: Political recruitment in twentieth-century Mexico.* Princeton University Press.

Solórzano, A. (1992). Sowing the seeds of neo-imperialism: The Rockefeller Foundation's yellow fever campaign in Mexico. *International Journal of Health Services*, 22(3), 529–554. https://doi.org/10.2190/XN07-TUVY-NKPT-WWP3.

Spalding, R. J. (1981). State power and its limits: Corporatism in Mexico. *Comparative Political Studies*, 14(2), 139–161.

Stallings, B. (1992). International influence on economic policy: Debt, stabilization, and structural reform. In S. Haggard & R. Kaufman (eds.), *The politics of economic adjustment: International constraints, distributive conflicts, and the state* (pp. 41–88). Princeton University Press.

Stavans, I. (2011). *José Vasconcelos: The prophet of race.* Rutgers University Press.

Transparency International (2018). Corruption Perceptions Index 2018. https://www.tra nsparency.org/files/content/pages/CPI_2018_Executive_Summary_EN.pdf.

Transparency International (n.d.). Anti-corruption glossary. https://www.transparency. org/glossary/term/political_corruption.

Vaughan, M. K. (1997). *Cultural politics in the revolution: Teachers, peasants, and schools in Mexico, 1930–1940*. The University of Arizona Press.

Vaughan, M. K. (2006). Nationalizing the countryside: Schools and rural communities in the 1930s. In M. K. Vaughan & S. E. Lewis (eds.), *The eagle and the virgin: Nation and cultural revolution in Mexico, 1920–1940* (pp. 157–175). Duke University Press.

Walker, L. E. (2013). *Waking from the dream: Mexico's middle classes after 1968*. Stanford University Press. https://ebookcentral-proquest-com.ezproxy.library.uq.edu.au/lib/ uql/detail.action?docID=1102616#.

Wences, L. (2018). Doctor Guillermo Soberón: Protagonista de la historia de la salud y la educación en México [Dr Guillermo Soberón: Key actor in the history of the Mexican health and education sectors]. Gaceta, Facultad de Medicina UNAM. http://gaceta.fa cmed.unam.mx/index.php/2018/11/22/doctor-guillermo-soberon-protagonista-de-la-historia-de-la-salud-y-la-educacion-en-mexico/.

Weston, C. H. (1983). The political legacy of Lázaro Cárdenas. *The Americas*, 39(3), 383–405. https://doi.org/10.2307/981231.

Zavaleta, N. (2020). Hallan ocho fosas clandestinas en Playa Vicente, Veracruz [Eight clandestine graves are found in Playa Vicente, Veracruz]. *Proceso*. https://www.proceso. com.mx/nacional/2020/12/7/hallan-ocho-fosas-clandestinas-en-playa-vicente-veracruz-254050.html.

Zolov, E. (2004). Showcasing the 'land of tomorrow': Mexico and the 1968 Olympics. *The Americas*, 61(2), 159–188. https://doi.org/10.1353/tam.2004.0195.

3 The Cultural Politics of Language in Obesity Policy

The practices around food that I observed in 2016 in schools in Veracruz, Mexico were, to a certain extent, shaped by four obesity policies launched between 2010 and 2014. The first of these policies was the Acuerdo Nacional contra la Salud Alimentaria (ANSA). Launched in January 2010, ANSA was a broad strategy proposing a range of more focalized initiatives to 'fight' obesity across different realms—the workplace, the household, the school. The only proposal which nonetheless materialized in policy was the *Lineamientos 2010*, a policy regulating food and promoting healthy eating in schools. In 2013 and 2014, ANSA and the *Lineamientos 2010* were, respectively, replaced by the Estrategia Nacional contra el Sobrepeso, la Obesidad y la Diabetes (ENSOD) and the *Lineamientos 2014*. This policy adjustment came after the federal administration running Mexico changed in 2012. These four policies are different in many respects, but they also share similarities. Notably, they are both underpinned by the 'healthy lifestyles' language: that is, as obesity preventive measures, they seek to educate individuals to make healthier food choices and to be physically active.[1]

This book argues that healthy lifestyles has worked to divert attention away from the political and economic roots of obesity, shifting the blame onto an 'uneducated' population, and to expand market interests in the name of 'health'. In Chapters 1 and 2, I explained how the market-driven trade and economic policies implemented from the 1980s have radically transformed the eating practices of the population in Mexico. I also described how the adoption of these same policies enabled—and indeed demanded—the re-orientation of how the health of the population was conceptualized, administered and researched. The dismantling of the welfare state coincided with the rise of a discourse of choice, which depicted people as rational decision makers who needed to insure themselves against risk. This transfer of the health sector from public to private hands was proposed based on the idea of increasing "quality" and "efficiency". Freedom to choose was a principle underlying privatization: people needed to have health care options and choose the best for them, rather than having access to only one public service. These ideas were seconded by powerful 'civil society organizations' that were created at the time. Heavily funded by corporations, organizations like FUNSALUD, for example, increased their capacity to shape health policy and the production (research and lobbying) and dissemination (professional organizations and tertiary education) of health knowledge.

DOI: 10.4324/9781003356264-3

Building upon this background, this chapter examines the language under-pinning ANSA, ENSOD and the two versions of the *Lineamientos* to show how obesity has been constructed as a problem of policy and why healthy lifestyles has been articulated and by whom. This analysis departs from the understanding of policy as a social and cultural construction where interests of all sorts, power dynamics and struggles over meaning are at stake. Policies therefore are not only technical constructions to address social problems; they are equally political. Poli-cies come to exist under specific contextual conditions, and they can also be used to channel different agendas as they are spoken about. Every word included in a policy document, for instance, is a highly symbolic device: they embody the poli-tical project of governments. The language of policies is never value-free. It is produced amidst struggles over meaning and relations of power. While multiple actors can have their say in policymaking, words, and the message they convey, can be traced to a particular locus of enunciation.[2]

The data set upon which this discussion is grounded comes primarily from policy documents, complemented by interviews conducted with policymakers in Mexico City in 2016 and reports.[3] I approach these altogether as discourse; that is, as a form of language framed by particular interests and knowledges that is intended to do something. Language does not exist outside of its producers. Language therefore carries multiple intentions. Written words within policy documents, which are part of the language of policy, are purposefully selected to frame a problem and its solutions in a particular way, which thereby implies that other views are left out. This chapter shows how the energy balance, shared responsibility and multifactorial discourses—and words associated to them, such as "healthy", "fight", "allies", "progress", "lifestyle", "diet", "education" and so on—have aided to transfer the responsibility of a structural problem into individual hands and to expand the interests of corporations.

Policies discursively construct subjects, spaces and practices. In ANSA, for example, it is assumed that *all* schools, and their communities, across Mexico are well resourced and that they have the time and willingness to promote healthy lifestyles. It is equally assumed that schools have the infrastructure, personnel and money needed to feed students. Chapters 4 and 5 challenge these depictions with empirical material from the day-to-day. But as starting point, this chapter pro-blematizes the way in which schools, members of the school community and food practices in schools are constructed by the language of anti-obesity policy.

In what follows, I first describe how obesity is framed as a problem and what solutions, and why, are proposed to 'fight' it. The analysis underpinning this dis-cussion focuses on how particular regimes of knowledge have validated the multi-factorial discourse as the explanation to obesity as an intrinsic outcome of 'progress' that needs to be addressed through individual lifestyle change. Second, I show how the discourses of energy balance and shared responsibility have facili-tated the corporatization of obesity policy and the deployment of narrow views on the relation between food and health. I then discuss why and how schools have been discursively constructed as anti-obesity sites, and the limitations of this view. I end this chapter claiming for the need of bringing culture into the making of obesity policy. Overall, the discussions in these chapter are informed by the discussions in Chapters 1 and 2 and are subsequently informing the discussions in Chapters 4, 5 and 6.

Knowledge and Power: Enunciating Solutions

Through ANSA, the Mexican government, corporations and NGOs reached consensus on the causes of the obesity problem and its solution. Part of the success of this agreement was the shared understanding that obesity results from an imbalance between energy consumed and energy spent, and that "unity" is fundamental to 'fight' obesity. The ten actions proposed in ANSA were framed by these logics. The proposed actions were focused on both individual behavioral change (through the provision of information) and on the regulation of the environment to facilitate healthy choices. However, not all the actions proposed were pursued through policy. The *Lineamientos 2010*, a policy to regulate food and promote healthy lifestyles in schools, was the only targeted policy that materialized from ANSA; probably because education-related anti-obesity policies are usually the least harmful to corporate interests.[4]

ANSA and the *Lineamientos 2010* had a relatively short life. In 2012, Enrique Peña Nieto won back the presidency of Mexico for the PRI. In 2013, the Peña Nieto administration launched ENSOD and the *Lineamientos 2014* to, respectively, replace ANSA and the *Lineamientos 2010*. One of the reasons why ENSOD was launched to substitute ANSA was because the latter "lacked" mechanisms to "coordinate the actions implemented by government agencies and the private sector" (p. 27). ENSOD was presented as a more robust framework with broader policy options and more accountability mechanisms to measure their success. Adolfo, the director of the NGO Anti-obesity Coalition, agreed with this point. During our interview in his office in Mexico City, he mentioned that ANSA had simply been a "list of good wishes" without a proper legal framework, funds or inter-sectorial collaboration. ENSOD filled these gaps by coordinating the deployment of actions across sectors. One of the most celebrated outcomes of this strategy was the creation of a levy on sugary drinks, snack foods and confectionery, known as the "sugar tax". This tax was intended to supplement the *Lineamientos 2014*, in particular around the provision of free, safe running water to drink in schools (for a discussion on this topic, see Chapter 6).

The two sets of policies mentioned above are distinct, but they also share a grounding rationale. Beyond some general nuances, the consistent framing of obesity and its solutions in both ANSA and ENSOD show how the same language underpins them. Risk, for example, is an intrinsic discourse in these strategies. In ANSA (p. 12), statistics are used to show that obesity "reduces workers' productivity", threatens the "stability of the health and pensions systems" and negatively impacts the household economy. This same point is made in ENSOD (pp. 7-8), where statistics are displayed to show the correlation between obesity and lower productivity among workers, which put the "development" of Mexico at risk. This discourse justifies the need for anti-obesity strategies. The "high prevalence of overweight and obesity [in Mexico]", it is stated in ANSA (p. 10), "represents a burning public health problem that requires the deployment of a national policy that can address the multifactorial nature of the problem". In a similar vein, in ENSOD (p. 7), it is highlighted that overweight and obesity "are complex and multifactorial problems" that need to be addressed through "coordinated actions from the public, private and civil society sectors".

The multifactorial discourse is also embedded in both strategies, as can be seen in the above statements. This discourse situates obesity as the result of multiple integrated factors across different realms. Factors such as migration, change in labor patterns, economic growth and technological development are said to, in some form, generate the conditions for obesity. The multifactorial discourse sits within a broader scientific view, the epidemiological transition model, that proposes that morbidity and mortality patterns have been continuously altered by "progress". This model has been used, together with the framework of the new public health, by health professionals with ties to FUNSALUD to delineate policy responses to noncommunicable diseases (NCDs).[5] Under this rationale, obesity is presented in both ANSA and ENSOD as an immanent outcome of modernity. In ANSA (pp. 16–17), for example, it is said that "change in food availability and consumption and the drastic change of lifestyles in a relatively short period of time" is mostly due to "economic growth", "urbanization" and "higher life expectancy". Similarly, in ENSOD (pp. 21–22) it is highlighted that obesity results from the "Westernization of the Mexican diet", mostly characterized by a wider consumption of ultra-processed products enabled by technological development, a reduction in cooking time and a higher purchasing power.

As this book has shown so far, all these factors are associated in some form to the increase in body weight Mexicans have experienced from the 1990s. Yet a problem with the multifactorial discourse is that it, like the epidemiolocal transition model itself, is underpinned by a linear and orderly view of "progress".[6] Furthermore, as Brown and Bell (2008) have argued, the application of this model to explain NCDs in Non-Western countries is problematic given that it has been developed with the view of "progress" that is associated with the West. Martínez-Salgado and Leal-Fernández (2003, p. 542, original emphasis) have claimed that the epidemiological transition "doctrine" has generated a constant "need for *more prevention*" which hides the pressure on the health system. This point is evident in the ENSOD (pp. 8–9) where it is stated that to face the negative health and economic consequences associated with obesity, the government urgently needs to change from the current "curative approach" to health care towards a "preventive model". Conceiving obesity as the result of multiple factors is not wrong in itself, yet it can obscure the political and economic roots of the problem.[7]

Diets, and the ways of managing the health of the population, have constantly changed, and "progress" has occurred in multiple forms throughout history. Economic growth, urbanization, technological innovation and the Westernization of diets and lifestyle, for example, were central tasks to the modernity project that policymakers pursued in post-revolutionary Mexico (Chapter 2). The transformation of forms of living is an ongoing project in Mexico. The argument that the body weight of Mexicans has dramatically increased due to the "progress" that Mexico has experienced from the 1980s is therefore only a partial explanation of the problem.

The "progress" stressed in ANSA and ENSOD has been accompanied by structural economic changes which have negatively affected the living and working conditions of a large section of the population. Diets and the forms of living among the Mexican population have not changed by magic. Actors with particular economic interests have set the conditions for these changes to occur. Power, politics and capital define how the ways of eating and living are transformed over a period of time. Mintz (1985, 2013) has offered powerful accounts of how the human allure to sugar has had more to do with imperial colonialism, global trade and the development of capitalism, than with the biochemical sensation that sweetness spawns in palates. In a similar way, the wider availability of ultra-processed products in Mexico only became possible after a series of political and economic decisions, taken in the name of the market, facilitated the expansion of corporations.

Yet the multifactorial discourse has aided to advance the idea that Mexicans have gained weight because of factors such as technological development, economic progress and changes in forms of living. But more important for the overall argument of this book is the fact that this discourse has also laid the ground for a more explicit participation of non-state entities in the management of the population's health and to attenuate any potential harm the policy may inflict on corporations. To further elaborate on this point, it is important to say that a discourse never acts independently of others. In this case, the multifactorial discourse is closely linked to those of energy balance and shared responsibility. In connection with the latter, the multifactorial discourse helps to dissociate one product (ultra-processed products) from being the main cause of obesity. The idea that obesity results from the sum of multiple factors has also reinforced the idea that solving obesity is a "shared responsibility" among sectors and actors. Intertwined, these discourses have facilitated the corporatization of obesity and healthy eating policies in Mexico.

Corporatizing Obesity Policy

In spite of the change from ANSA to ENSOD triggered by the presidential transition of 2012, three points remained central in the obesity policy agenda in Mexico. First, the framing of obesity as a multifactorial problem which is intrinsic to "progress". Second, given its multifactorial nature, the 'fight' against obesity needs to be fought in collaboration. Third, although ENSOD widened the scope of anti-obesity actions proposed in ANSA, it also emphasized the regulation of food and the promotion of healthy eating in schools as one of its central solutions to obesity.

The making of policy is a complex process where multiple voices are heard, and myriad interests are at play. In the case of obesity policy, researchers, government officials, activists, the 'civil society' and corporations have spoken about obesity and its solutions. Yet not all these voices materialized equally in policy.[8] This section describes how the language of obesity policy has been significantly shaped by, and for the benefit of, corporations. This is what I refer to as the "corporatization of policy".

The multifactorial discourse framed obesity as inherent with "progress", given the general improvement of life conditions among the population. Through this discourse obesity is seen as the result of multiple factors, yet obesity policy has primarily focused only on two of them: food and physical activity. From the start of the obesity debate in Mexico in the early 2000s, these two factors became the focus of intervention. Food was conceptualized as "energy intake"—as pure nutrients with a concrete biological function—and physical activity as the mechanism through which energy could "burned". This energy balance discourse is at the core of obesity policy.

The launching of ANSA in 2010 officialized the 'fight' against obesity. Yet the language underpinning it started to frame the obesity debate in Mexico from 2006. Before ANSA, several anti-obesity initiatives led by food and drink corporations were at work. In 2006, for example, PepsiCo launched its healthy lifestyles program, Vive Saludable [Living Healthy] and Walmart launched Juego y Comida [Play and Food]. One year later, Coca-Cola launched Movimiento Bienestar [Movement and Wellness] and Nestlé released Nutrir: Niños Saludables [Nutrir: Healthy Kids]. As the names of these initiatives suggest, obesity was framed as an energy balance problem resulting from poor eating choices and an inactive lifestyle.[9]

Likewise, the energy balance discourse permeated the discussion of anti-obesity policy proposals in the Mexican Congress between 2006 and 2009. In 2007, for instance, a motion to regulate the marketing of ultra-processed products to children was rejected. Opponents to the proposal, who had corporate ties, argued that it violated the "freedom of trade" underwritten by NAFTA, was detrimental for the national economy and unfairly "stigmatized" ultra-processed products. The problem, they stated, was not the consumption of these products, but people's lack of nutritional knowledge and unwillingness to be physically active. The solution, therefore, was not "prohibition" but to "educate" people to have a "healthy lifestyle" (Diario de los Debates [Diary of debates], 2007).

It is then not unsurprising why the *Lineamientos 2010* was the only ANSA proposal that materialized in policy. The energy balance discourse notably shaped the language adopted to talk about school food and how it should be regulated in the name of 'fighting' obesity. An example of how corporations drew on this discourse both to frame anti-obesity policies and to protect their economic interests from the potential negative effects of these policies is observable in the making of the *Lineamientos 2010*.

In June 2010, when the first draft of this policy was released for public discussion, various corporations and businesses organizations expressed their discontent towards the policy draft's proposals. For example, ConMéxico, an influential businesses association, released a communiqué signed by its Executive President, Jaime Zabludovsky, an economist from Yale and Mexican deputy chief negotiator of NAFTA, claiming that the proposed definition of low-nutritional food and the association between this kind of food and obesity were mistaken. Obesity, the influential business association claimed, could not be attributed to particular foods but to the "imbalance between the energy intake, through food consumption, and energy expenditure, through physical activity" (ConMéxico, 2010).

BIMBO, a Mexican transnational bakery corporation, also released a communiqué claiming that banning ultra-processed products in school cooperatives, as the *Lineamientos 2010* draft proposed, was erroneous because obesity had multiple causes beyond food. Tying together the shared responsibility and the energy balance discourses, BIMBO claimed that to "fight" the problem "effectively" it was required that "all the stakeholders participate actively and constantly" to change the "eating habits and increasing the levels of physical activity and education" among Mexicans (BIMBO, 2010). In a similar line of critique, Coca-Cola México claimed that this policy draft was "skewed" because it was not supported by "strong scientific evidence". In a more direct connection to the energy balance discourse, the corporation stated that the draft of the *Lineamientos 2010* "stigmatize[d] products and ingredients" instead of "promoting healthy nutrition". Expressing their will to share the responsibility in tackling obesity, Coca-Cola México manifested their disposition to support actions conducted by the federal education authority to "promote the consumption of water as a healthy habit" and to "promote physical activity and sports" (Coca-Cola de México, 2010).

Further opposition against the policy draft was expressed in economic terms. Similar to the arguments used to block potentially harmful policy proposals in Congress, corporations and business associations claimed that the *Lineamientos 2010* would have a negative impact on the economy if passed as they were. After a heated consultation process, the *Lineamientos 2010* was redrafted and released in August 2010. Several modifications were made, many of which, as some have argued, weakened the scope of the *Lineamientos 2010* and made it more corporate-friendly (Charvel et al., 2015; Moise et al., 2011). Reading the policy document against this background shows the extent to which the energy balance discourse has been pushed by, and aided the interests of, corporations.

The energy balance discourse rests upon a conceptualization of food as a nutritional object with a particular biological aim that can be measured and used to govern. As I discuss in the next section, this view predominates the language of the *Lineamientos*. There is not anything necessarily wrong with this. Yet this technical language, as Chapter 5 demonstrates, is in constant tension with the cultural, political and economic conditions surrounding the social life of food in schools. This is why energy balance helps to shift the blame for obesity and reproduce narrow ideas between food, movement and bodily health. Gard and Wright (2005, p. 38) have argued that the energy-in/energy-out model lies on a "mechanistic thinking" that assumes that the body is "predictable and obeys laws that are more or less universal across time and space". After discussing empirical uncertainties within the literature, the authors claim that this model is problematic not only because it "produces untrue knowledge", but because in "the end, the question of what is 'true' about the causes and consequences of overweight and obesity will probably prove to be immaterial. The important questions [...] will probably be political, cultural and social" (p. 67).

In my time in schools in 2016, I observed the energy balance discourse materialized in plates, posters, puppets and cookbooks. Most of these objects—if not all—were brought into schools by corporate-sponsored healthy lifestyles programs. Their goal was to convey the food-as-energy message and thereby to make children aware of the need for measuring the energy consumed. Drawing upon the premise that 'fighting' obesity is a shared responsibility, these programs were designed as "public–private partnerships"; a mode of policy implementation widely encouraged from the beginning of the obesity debate and central to the actions proposed in both ANSA and ENSOD.

The phrase "Tackling Overweight and Obesity is a Shared Responsibility", for instance, appears in bold letters at the end of ANSA's conclusion. The phrase is a central reminder of what is stressed across the document: solving obesity requires "the collaboration of the most relevant actors from the public sector, businesses, the society, and the academy to develop policy and set accountability mechanisms" (pp. 24–42). The same language is used in ENSOD to justify the need for inter-sector "allies" and public–private partnerships. "This Strategy", states the Introduction of ENSOD (p. 9), "promotes the construction of national policy between the public, private and civil society sectors with the aim of generating healthy [*saludable*] eating and physical activity habits among the Mexican population".

The shared responsibility discourse has facilitated the corporatization of obesity policy in various interrelated ways. First, this discourse has made corporations indispensable actors in addressing obesity, justifying why programs that embody their own views on the relation between food and health are needed in schools. In conjunction with the multifactorial discourse, shared responsibility has also aided to downplay the negative impact ultra-processed products have had on the health of the population. Corporations have been extensively invested in dis-associating themselves and their products from being one of the main reasons for the obesity problem in Mexico. Shared responsibility has aided this goal, spreading the responsibility for the problem across multiple actors and realms. This discourse has also depicted the 'fight' against obesity as a democratic process in which not only government and business are involved, but also where "civil society" has a voice.

Yet what the shared responsibility discourse masks is that many of the 'civil society organizations' that have been given voice in the making of policy have deep corporate ties. If readers cast their minds back to Chapter 2, it will be recalled that the political transformation Mexico has undergone since the 1980s facilitated the emergence of myriad civil society organizations across multiple spaces. This process was seen fundamental in the democratization of Mexico, since the all-powerful regime that ruled Mexico for more than 70 years was made more accountable. However, as I described though FUNSALUD's case, civil society organizations, or NGOs, have complex politics and they can also be used to channel interests that are not necessarily for the public good (see Kamat, 2004).

In the obesity policy context, the civil society sector has been presented as an independent entity that represents neither government nor corporate interests, but those of the general population. This allusion is not necessarily wrong. As part of the research supporting this book, I interviewed three members of two NGOs that have been pro-actively wrestling corporate influence in obesity policymaking and arguing for policies that go beyond the usual behavioral change approach. The important role these NGOs—which I introduce in more detail in Chapter 6—have had in counteracting corporate power was also acknowledge by the nutrition researcher I interviewed. Yet, overall, in the language of policy "civil society" has been captured by market interests.

And here a distinction between ANSA and ENSOD needs to be highlighted. Both strategies, as I quoted above, draw upon shared responsibility to justify the need for the involvement of state and non-state actors in obesity policy. However, ENSOD goes far beyond this call. Across the document, the need for public–private partnership is emphasized and 'civil society organizations' with corporate ties are explicitly mentioned. On page 62 of this document, for instance, it is stressed that "partnerships with civil society organizations like Queremos Mexicanos Activos A.C. and Dar la Vuelta A.C." should be established to promote physical activity.

Dar la Vuelta [Let's Ride] was launched in 2011 by Nestlé as an initiative to promote healthy lifestyles. In 2016, Dar la Vuelta evolved into an 'independent' NGO, still funded by Nestlé, promoting "cycling, healthy lifestyles, physical activity" and had established "alliances" with local governments and the "Mexican Industry of Coca-Cola" (Darlavuelta, n.d.). Queremos Mexicanos Activos [We Want Active Mexicans] started as an NGO in 2012 with the aim of "activating", promoting physical activity, among the Mexican population (MexicanosActivos, n.d.).[10]

Both Queremos Mexicanos Activos and Dar la Vuelta were part of MOVISA, a broad network of NGOs, corporations and lobby groups sponsored by, or related to, corporations. MOVISA, which stands for Movimiento por una Vida Saludable [Movement for a Healthy Life], is "a comprehensive platform of communication and action that promotes healthy lifestyles". MOVISA was a powerful lobbyist strategy precisely because of the wide nature of its members: its list of "allies" includes banks, business organizations, media outlets and food and drink corporations (MOVISA, n.d.).[11] MOVISA was one of the most influential actors shaping ENSOD, and the subsequent obesity discussion in Mexico (Calvillo & Székely, 2018). The importance of these organizations in corporatizing obesity lies, of course, not only on their influence in shaping policy, but also in implementing it. Alone or in partnership with a government entity, corporate-sponsored NGOs or programs have been deployed in schools. It was under this shared responsibility discourse that Nestlé's "Eatwell Plate" entered into Emiliano Zapata Primary School (see Chapter 4).

In the section where the institutions framing and endorsing ENSOD are listed in the policy document, FUNSALUD is recorded as being "actively participating in preventing childhood obesity through research and the promotion of healthy eating and exercising habits" (ENSOD, p. 90). Apart from its role in shaping ENSOD, FUNSALUD also validated corporate-sponsored healthy eating strategies like that of Nestlé's global strategy—Healthy Kids. Between 1988 and 2018, as a stakeholder in central health policy, FUNSALUD's power spanned several actions and realms, including the designation of the Mexican secretary of health (see Chapter 2). Indeed, when ENSOD was released, the head of the Secretaría de Salud (SSA), Mercedes Juan, had moved into this position from her office as FUNSALUD's director.

However, Mexico is not the only country where obesity policy has been captured by corporations. The corporatization of obesity policy, and thereby healthy eating policies, is a global phenomenon. Scholars from across disciplines have demonstrated this point, which has assisted in increasing the awareness of corporate tactics to shape policy.[12] Yet a point that is somewhat absent from the conversation is that corporate interference with decision making in health was facilitated by the adoption of neoliberalism at a global scale, which transformed the way in which international governing bodies, such as the World Health Organization (WHO), framed policy and acted upon global health problems. From the 1980s, as critical health scholars have claimed, the WHO prioritized policies proposing market-driven solutions, which aimed more at contributing to economic growth than to social development and fostered the "partnerships" language (Chorev, 2012, 2013; Navarro, 2007, 2008). Thus, it is of no surprise that the multifactorial, energy balance and shared responsibility discourses are originally a WHO creation.[13]

The shared responsibility discourse has validated the emergence of organizations such as Queremos Mexicanos Activos, Dar la Vuelta and MOVISA as key actors to promote healthy lifestyles among Mexicans. These organizations have been used by corporations, businesses associations and neoliberal enthusiasts to channel their agendas disguised as "civil society" proposals. The extent to which these organizations have contributed to make 'healthy' Mexicans will probably remain unknown. However, they have been active advocates of other discourses that, framed by, and for the benefit of, corporations, have served to blame Mexicans for their unwillingness to be 'healthy'. At the heart of Queremos Mexicanos Activos, Dar la Vuelta and MOVISA, as their names lucidly suggest, lies the idea that a healthy lifestyle can be achieved if people are educated to maintain a balance between the energy that they consume and the energy they expend.

The *Lineamientos*: Emergence of a New Form of Governing School Food

ANSA proposed ten actions to 'fight' obesity. With some differences, mainly in terms of their targeted audience (e.g., breastfeeding mothers or school children), these actions are underpinned by the same rationale: Mexicans need to be educated to eat healthy and to be more physically active. To achieve these goals, multiple government entities are deemed crucial. However, schools receive a particular emphasis. This is graphically illustrated in the cover of ANSA, where cheerful students running on a school patio appear on the cover photo. ENSOD, as I described above, proposed actions beyond the school context, but it also suggested that the strategy was "particularly [directed] towards school-aged students".

Globally, schools have been made responsible for creating the childhood obesity problem. In line with the global obesity discussion (Swinburn et al., 1999), Mexican schools have been depicted in ANSA and ENSOD as "obesogenic environments".[14] This conceptualization has derived from research arguing that schools facilitate the conditions for children to gain body weight, mainly due to the high amounts of "junk food" children can access within schools. In ANSA (p. 17, emphasis added), for example, it is claimed that an "obesogenic environment prevails in *all* the schools around the country" because:

- Students can eat up to 5 times in 4½ hours in the school. The caloric intake during school time can be around half of the caloric requirements for the whole day (840 to 1259 kcal)
- There is a high availability of energetically dense foods
- Most of the children buy food in the school instead of bringing a snack from home
- The access to drinkable water is limited
- The availability of fruits and vegetables is low
- The break and the physical education lesson are the only opportunities that children have to do physical activity
- There is only one physical education lesson per week, and it lasts only 39 minutes in average. Children only have 9 minutes of moderate or intense physical activity, which shows the low quality of the class …

This construction of Mexican schools as obesogenic environments justified the pertinency of changing the way in which food practices were regulated in schools. Before the *Lineamientos 2010* were released, the production, sale and consumption of food had been ruled by the same policy for nearly 30 years, the *Reglamento 1982*. The language used to speak of food and to administer it was significantly different under this earlier policy. It required schools to create a cooperativa escolar [school cooperative], a committee of teachers, students and parents, to manage the production and sale of food in the school. With the cuts in public spending on education that began in the 1980s, food sales became a central income for the workings of schools. However, the *Lineamientos 2010* eliminated the cooperative model of organizing school food. Instead, it proposed that external vendors would be invited to tender and the winner would become the school food provider.[15] The *Lineamientos 2010* also introduced concepts such as "calories", "energy", "nutrients", "healthy", "unhealthy", "choice", etc. as terminologies for speaking of food and eating in schools. The main difference between the *Lineamientos 2010* and the *Reglamento 1982* is that the latter was focused on the economic organization of food sales in schools, whereas the former takes school food to be a tool of government with the purpose of making 'healthy' citizens (see Chapter 2). For this endeavor, a new language to speak about food in schools and the imperative of promoting healthy lifestyles through schools was introduced by the *Lineamientos 2010* (p. 4, emphasis added):

[O]besity and overweight are complex challenges in Mexico, and therefore, to face them it is required to develop and strengthen a new health culture. The school is the space par excellence where future citizens acquire the competencies to construct their own development and to *actively* and *responsibly* participate in their community. For this reason, schooling needs to be an integrating tool where health education is put into practice and curriculum content is developed by teachers to emphasize the importance of adopting healthy lifestyles, to encourage the self-care of one's health and to promote disease prevention.

Thus, the *dispositif of healthy lifestyles* has discursively produced schools as spaces for 'fighting' obesity. The release of the *Lineamientos 2010* as the new form of regulating school food as an imperative of health represented a historical break in the Mexican education system. From the launch of the first *Reglamento* in 1932, the management of food in schools remained, at least on paper, almost the same until 2010. The *Lineamientos 2010*, however, sparked the attention of what was prepared, sold and consumed in schools, which triggered a variety of new dynamics (Treviño Ronzón & Sánchez Pacheco, 2014). This book shows the workings of these dynamics from the day-to-day of two schools. While I consider that a change in the regulation of school food was required, the way in which this shift was done created the conditions for the expansion of neoliberal logics in the name of health. With the idea that Mexican students need to *actively* and *responsibly* take care of their health to prevent obesity, for example, the makers of this policy transferred the responsibility of obesity from a macro-structural problem into an individual lifestyle matter.

Schools are complex spaces. Within their walls, curriculum delivery intersects with politics and myriad policies. The history outlined in Chapter 2, for instance, showed us the role that schools, teachers and education policy had in the creation of a 'modern' Mexico. In public health terms, schools have been historically endowed with the responsibility of 'solving' different health-related issues affecting societies. However, while they can reach intimate spaces that no other social institution can, the extent in which schools can 'solve' public health problems is rather limited (Gard & Pluim, 2014). This is especially the case if schools are under-resourced and caught up in complex party and union politics, as in Mexico.

In 2014, the *Lineamientos 2014* replaced the *Lineamientos 2010*, almost immediately after ENSOD substituted ANSA. In a general sense, both versions of the *Lineamientos* seek to regulate the food and to promote healthy eating in schools. However, one important difference between these policies can be seen in the roles assigned to teachers. In the 2010 document, for instance, the word "teacher(s)" appears 16 times.[16] Beyond the abstract number, what is compelling is that in the *Lineamientos 2010* (p. 12), teachers were highlighted as key policy actors in improving the health status of Mexican children given that they were "promoters, coordinators and direct agents in the learning process". Teachers are depicted not only as professionals, but also as political agents belonging to a union. The teachers' union and education policy go hand to hand in Mexico. For instance, it has been argued that the political support of the Sindicato Nacional de Trabajadores de la Educación (SNTE) [Mexican National Teachers Union] was key for the narrow triumph of Felipe Calderón in the elections of 2006 (Larreguy et al., 2017; Ornelas, 2008). Consequently, the SNTE gained a great leverage capacity to shape education policy in the 2006–2012 administration (Ornelas, 2012).

However, the central role given to teachers in the *Lineamientos 2010* was downsized in the *Lineamientos 2014*. In this latter policy, teachers are mentioned only once in a borderline comment on page 4. Teachers were even obliterated from the definition of "school community" included in the glossary (p. 3). Making teachers absent from the school community definition in the *Lineamientos 2014* might appear a small issue. However, this small change in the policy language reflects the change that the 2013 Education Reform introduced into the Mexican education system at large. Championed as one the most important reforms launched by the Peña Nieto administration, perhaps just behind the energy reform (see Chapter 2), the 2013 Education Reform introduced deep changes in the management of the Mexican education system, both at the government and the union levels. These changes were perceived by teachers as detrimental for teachers' rights and public education itself (Levinson, 2014; López Aguilar, 2013). Indeed, the *Lineamientos 2014* strengthened the punitive language against teachers if schools do not comply with the policy. The place that teachers are assigned in both versions of the *Lineamientos* also reflects the less 'educative' and more regulatory nature of the *Lineamientos* 2014. This might explain why the substitution of the *Lineamientos 2010* for the 2014 version went almost unnoticed by the teachers and the education authorities that I talked to for this research.

The two *Lineamientos* propose the regulation of school food to be the key ingredient for making 'healthy' Mexicans. For instance, both the *Lineamientos 2010* (p. 8) and the *Lineamientos 2014* (p. 3) contain a section entitled, "Title II: On the Configuration of Students' Correct Diet", where the "principles" of a "correct diet" are listed. Visibly underpinned by the energy balance discourse, these principles demand that schools offer to students a diet that is "complete", "equilibrated" and "varied", "innocuous" and, of course, "*saludable*". Through this language, the *Lineamientos* have deployed the discursive arrangements that have constructed food as a tool of government conceptualized in terms of nutrients, calories, portions and energy. The cultural and political dimension around food practices is obliterated.

While in general terms the language across them is quite similar, there are specificities within the text that tell us interesting things about the degree in which the neoliberal form of government was made material in these two policy documents. A simple, but highly illustrative example comes from word and tense choice. In the two versions of the *Lineamientos*, after the desired principles of a "correct diet" are listed, a sentence stresses the role of schools in enabling student access to a "correct" diet:

Based on the principles described in this section, in schools it will be promoted: (*Lineamientos 2010*, p. 8)Based on the principles described in this section, schools:(*Lineamientos 2014*, p. 4)

In the first sentence, from the *Lineamientos 2010*, the use of "promote" in future tense shows that this policy did not assume that schools could provide students with a "good" diet just by themselves. Instead, the selection of this verb denotes that schools can make "correct" diets available for students *if* they are assisted by other entities in creating favorable circumstances for this to happen. In contrast, the absence of any verb after "schools" in the sentence from the *Lineamientos 2014* shows that the writers of this policy document endowed schools with the responsibility of facilitating "correct" diets, without saying that other entities are required for this enterprise to be accomplished. This point can probably be better understood if we consider that private interests had an even stronger foothold in shaping this policy than they had in 2010, when the *Lineamientos* were initially released.

Beyond their differences, which can be measured in terms of the penetration of private interests in their shaping, the *Lineamientos 2010* and the *Lineamientos 2014* share the same ultimate goal: decrease the energy intake of students within schools. Implicitly, the *Lineamientos'* construction of schools as anti-obesity sites assumes that schools are well-funded and have the required infrastructure (playing fields and kitchens, for example) and materials to promote healthy lifestyles. This might be true in some Western countries from where the idea of schools as anti-obesity sites has been taken (Story, 1999; Story et al., 2009), but this is not always the case in most public schools in Mexico.

Other assumptions are that the school staff have the knowledge about, and the time for, doing health promotion work. Families are imagined without class disparities. Schools have been presented as de-politicized spaces: they are envisaged as spaces where pedagogy and curriculum delivery are the most important and the only tasks. These assumptions are naive. Many public schools in the country lack resources and infrastructure and are usually attended by the poor and working and lower-middle class students. Also, the Mexican education system is a highly politicized environment. Education departments, school districts and schools are entrenched between the teachers' union politics, the state government's politics, the local community's politics and the school's own politics. Nonetheless, these important issues were silenced across both versions of the *Lineamientos*. I will return to this discursive construction in Chapters 4, 5 and 6.

Bringing Culture into Policy

Every word included in a policy document is a highly symbolic device: they embody political projects of government. Therefore, policies are political constructions in themselves. The language underpinning the four policies discussed in this chapter has served to transfer to people's hands the responsibility of ensuring themselves against the health risks that come with a globalized, market-driven economy.

This point can be seen in the word choice in the policies. "Families and individuals", ANSA (p. 40, emphasis added) stresses, "*must* have a better knowledge of the relationship between nutrition, physical activity, weight and health to *take better decisions* about their diet and physical activity levels". With small differences, ENSOD (p. 46, emphasis added) also accentuates that Mexicans "*need* to have a better health education to be able to *make the best food choices* for a balanced diet and a proper energy intake". The use of the verbs *must* and *need* expresses a command for Mexican families and individuals to adopt 'healthier lifestyles'. Implicit in these commands is the idea that *all* Mexican families have both the time and the resources to acquire the 'knowledge' about dieting and exercising that is required to take 'good choices'. Nonetheless, this visualization of how families are resourced—that emerged from the theorization of urban, middle-class policymakers trained in a US-based approach to public health and corporations—is not completely connected with the material conditions under which millions of families live.

According to the OECD (n.d.-b), for example, the real minimum wages in Mexico are the lowest among the OECD countries. In 2016, the year in which I conducted fieldwork, the real minimum annual salary in Mexico was $2,058.3 USD.[17] Mexican households, considering the income of two adults, have an average income of between two and three times the minimum wage (INEGI, 2018). These considerably low wages, which negatively impact a household's purchasing power (Moreno-Brid, Garry, & Krozer, 2016; Moreno-Brid et al., 2016), dramatically contrast with the high number of hours that Mexican people work to make their income. Mexico ranks first in the OECD's 'Average annual hours actually worked per worker' list. In 2018, workers from Mexico worked an average of 2,148 hours, well above average of 1,734 hours for other OECD countries (OECD, n.d.-a).[18] These are some of the tangible effects of the neoliberalism *à la mexicaine*.

Thus, with those data in mind, it would have been fairer to state in these policy documents that Mexican families and individuals *must* or *need* to be provided with *more optimal*—or less unfavorable—*conditions* to be able to make good eating and exercising choices. Saying this, I want to emphasize that, in most cases, people do not lack the knowledge to make 'healthy choices'. Instead, as I will demonstrate in Chapters 4 and 5, what they lack is time and money. Therefore, it should not be a surprise that under this context, policies telling Mexicans to "eat better" and "move more" may become empty words, even if they are robustly based on the best evidence available.

Obesity policy discursively constructs food in terms of nutrients, portions and energy that need to be measured in the name of health, and depicts the school as the space par excellence to channel this view. This discourse that presents food-as-energy has permeated into health promotion work and in the practices around food in schools. The cooks in the fieldwork stories narrated in Chapter 1, for instance, were the object of this discourse, yet they resisted and adapted it in multiple ways.

The aim of this chapter was twofold. First, it exposed how the language of policy has been significantly framed by narrow corporate views of health and food and their relation to health. Second, it has shown how this language served the expansion of market—read corporate—interests.

The making of ANSA, ENSOD and the *Lineamientos* was of course complex. Multiple actors, most of them well-intentioned and committed to health equity, pushed more comprehensive views on what to do with obesity. Yet their capacity to shape, and put to work, discourse was not as central as that of corporations as a result of the power that is bestowed upon them by money and political influence. One of the main gaps in obesity policy is precisely its lack of a cultural perspective on how food, health and bodies are intertwined beyond bio-medical discourses in the complex day-to-day. This is why Chapter 5 shows how the cultured and historical dimensions of food have allowed the articulation of a material resistance against 'healthy lifestyles' through the practice of *cooking* in schools.

School food regulations are needed. Yet their current narrow, biologist framing together with the complexity of the education system and the material conditions under which many families live in Mexico, make the aims of these policies hard to be achieved. What Mexico needs to confront the public health problem posed by obesity are structural policies to improve the quality of life (e.g., better salaries, more leisure time) and the access to food. My use of "structural" requires some clarification here.

For some, the sugar tax that has been in place since 2014 and the food labelling that was passed in 2019 are structural policies since they are aimed at modifying the "environment". These policies are indisputably important in protecting the nutritional health of the population. Yet they are also underpinned by the choice discourse, which assumes individuals to be rational decision-makers whose consumption of ultra-processed products can be disincentivized through economic penalties and more information. The sugar tax and food labels, however, do not address the conditions that enable the existence and consumption of these products.

Following Gálvez (2018) and Otero (2018), I hence suggest obesity in Mexico should be addressed by both individual-level solutions focusing on behavior change in combination with policies aimed at reverting the negative effects market-drive policies have had over food systems. Revising trade agreements, re-introducing tariffs for agricultural commodities in the global market and revitalizing low-scale agricultural production, for instance, may do more to improve diets of Mexicans than simply telling them that they need to eat healthy. However, education-related policies are, of course, more politically viable policies, which explains the direction the government has taken to date (see also Gard, 2010; Gard & Wright, 2005).

Conclusion

In Mexico, obesity has become a public health issue amidst the change in food practices enabled by the adoption of neoliberalism as a form of government. The body weight of Mexicans started to increase considerably from the late 1980s due to the wider availability and consumption of sugary drinks and ultra-processed foods facilitated by economic policy shifts like NAFTA. ANSA, ENSOD, the *Lineamientos 2010* and the *Lineamientos 2014*, I have claimed here, were released to ameliorate, from a public health perspective, a problem that has deep political and economic roots. This is not something necessarily bad. Indeed, social policy should, ideally, amend, or at least lessen, the side effects of "progress". However, under neoliberalism, policies such as the ones I have interrogated here have been used to expand the rule of the market over society to shape subjectivities aligned with the neoliberal project. In this chapter I have argued that these four policies have, partially, accomplished these tasks.

Deploying an analysis focused on both the macro and the micro features of discourse and on the interactions between them, I interrogated ANSA, ENSOD and the two *Lineamientos* to shed light on how particular forces and regimes of knowledge have validated the promotion of healthy lifestyles, particularly through schools, as *the* obesity solution. These documents portray scientific and political debates. In the process of making these policies some voices prevailed over others and this is tangible in the language used in these four documents. I showed how political and economic forces appealing to the neoliberal project have validated a particular public health knowledge that has framed obesity as an intrinsic outcome of progress that needs to be fought through 'educating' Mexican people in what and how they should eat. Therefore, these policies have been released to shape rational subjects who take care of themselves, regardless of the adverse conditions that neoliberalism has provoked. My central argument in this chapter was that, although there were multiple voices in the process, in the end neoliberal enthusiasts and corporations have prevailed in crafting the language of policy.

Encouraging Mexicans to adopt healthy lifestyles to avoid obesity sounds contradictory when about a half of the population lives in poverty (CONEVAL, 2016); wages are very low and Mexican workers work the most hours annually out of all OECD countries. This is a different reality compared to the one in Western countries where these solutions have emerged, and basically been copied from. Through Chapters 4 and 5, I will show what happens when the myriad discourses that have emerged around obesity and its solutions meet the everyday lives of schools.

Notes

1 For simplicity, I will only add the page number to the documents when using material from them. For example: ANSA (p. 1), ENSOD (p. 1), *Lineamientos 2010* (p. 1). These sources appear in the list of references as: ANSA (2010), ENSOD (2013), *Lineamientos 2010*, and *Lineamientos 2014*.
2 Vallgårda's (2015a, 2015b, 2022) approach to the study of obesity policy has influenced my analysis in this chapter.
3 For a clarification of my treatment of "policymakers", see footnote 7 in Chapter 1.
4 One nutrition researcher and one member of one of the NGOs emphasized this point during our interviews. Early drafts of the *Lineamientos 2010* though did face fierce opposition from corporations. These proposals were said to be against trade rules and harmful for the economy. As a result, the final version of this policy was modified to be more corporate-friendly (Charvel, Cobo, & Hernandez-Avila, 2015). Vallgårda (2015a), Gard (2010) and Gard and Wright (2005) also discuss this point.
5 For examples, see Frenk (2006); Frenk, Bobadilla, Sepúlveda, & Cervantes (1989); Frenk, Bobadilla, Stern, Frejka, & Lozano (1991); Frenk, Frejka, et al. (1991).

6 In this regard, Brown and Bell (2008) have argued that there is danger in uncritically adopting this model to explain NCDs in the Third World because it implies that these countries have mirrored the patterns of "progress", and therefore the emergence of NCDs derived from "progress", in First World countries.

7 Martínez-Salgado and Leal-Fernández (2003, p. 544) further argue that the epidemiological transition model "says nothing of the complex balance between morbidity and mortality, or of their relationship to the specific constellations from which they have arisen".

8 For examples of how corporations have shaped/driven obesity policy in Mexico, see Calvillo & Székely (2018); Charvel, Cobo & Hernandez-Avila (2015); Gómez (2019); Moise, Cifuentes, Orozco & Willet (2011); Monterrosa et al. (2015).

9 This message was emphasized during the launching of these initiatives, which were implemented in partnership with the national education authority, the SEP. See PepsiCo (2006) and (Vázquez Mota, 2007a, 2007b).

10 Queremos Mexicanos Activos's website has constantly changed since the first time I accessed it in late 2015. The link provided will direct the reader to the current version of the website.

11 I accessed MOVISA's website in February 2020 the last time. In August 2020, I tried to access the site again, but it was "under construction".

12 Greenhalgh (2016, 2019, 2021) shows the pivotal role the International Life Science Institute (ILSI) has had in aiding Coca-Cola to largely shape obesity policy in China. Lougheed (2006), Mialon et al. (2021) and Nestle (2015) have also show how ILSI has shaped policy for the benefit of corporations.

13 The technical report *Obesity: Preventing and Managing the Global Epidemic* was the first global institutional statement regarding the obesity problem (WHO, 2000). Four years later, the WHO's *Global Strategy on Diet, Physical Activity and Health* (WHO, 2004) was launched.

14 Guthman (2011) claims that the obesogenic environments thesis rests on a narrow association between food availability and consumption, physical inactivity and body weight in which people are depicted as passive subjects over whom the context imposes its rules without agency on behalf the subjects. For a critique of the schools-as-obesogenic-environments idea, see Tenorio (2022).

15 This was a common practice already happening in schools before 2010, mostly due to the inoperability of the *Reglamento 1982* for multiple reasons, but this practice became then official. See Chapter 5.

16 In Spanish, teacher is translated as "*maestro*" for males and "*maestra*" for women. The word "*docente*", which refers both to male and women, is a synonym of teacher. The counting made here includes the words: "*maestros*" (6), "*maestras*" (1), "*docentes*" (6) and "*docente*" (3).

17 To have a point of comparison, in the same year, the countries with the highest minimum wages were Luxembourg (25,385.8 USD), Netherlands (24,741.1 USD) and Australia (23,915.4 USD). Even the countries that share the bottom of the list with Mexico have a considerably higher minimum wage: Russia (3,080.4 USD), Brazil (4,872.0 USD) and Chile (6,682.2 USD).

18 In the countries with the highest minimum wages, workers worked considerably less hours in 2018: Luxembourg 1,506 hours, Netherlands 1,431 hours, and Australia 1,723 hours.

References

Acuerdo Nacional para la Salud Alimentaria. Estrategia contra el sobrepeso y la obesidad [National Agreement for Nutritional Health. Strategy against overweight and obesity] (ANSA) (2010). Secretaría de Salud, México.

BIMBO (2010). *Opinión Lineamientos para expendio o distribución de alimentos y bebidas en planteles (B001002707).* http://187.191.71.192/expediente/8623/recibido/366/B001002707.

Brown, T., & Bell, M. (2008). Imperial or postcolonial governance? Dissecting the genealogy of a global public health strategy. *Social Science & Medicine, 67*(10), 1571–1579. https://doi.org/10.1016/j.socscimed.2008.07.027.

Calvillo, A., & Székely, A. (2018). *La trama oculta de la epidemia: obesidad, industria alimentaria y conflicto de interés* [*The epidemic's hidden story: Obesity, corporations and conflicts of interest*]. El Poder del Consumidor.

Charvel, S., Cobo, F., & Hernández-Ávila, M. (2015). A process to establish nutritional guidelines to address obesity: Lessons from Mexico. *Journal of Public Health Policy, 36* (4), 426–439. https://doi.org/10.1057/jphp.2015.28.

Chorev, N. (2012). *The World Health Organization between North and South.* Cornell University Press.

Chorev, N. (2013). Restructuring neoliberalism at the World Health Organization. *Review of International Political Economy, 20*(4), 627–666. https://doi.org/10.1080/09692290.2012.690774.

Coca-Cola de México (2010). (B001002395). Letter sent to COFEMER in response to the first draft of the *Lineamientos 2010,* during the consultation process. Available from the author on request.

CONEVAL (2016). Medición de la pobreza. Pobreza en México. Resultados de pobreza en México 2016 a nivel nacional y por entidades federativas [Measuring poverty in Mexico in 2016 at the federal and state levels]. Consejo Nacional de Evaluación de la Política de Desarrollo Social (CONEVAL). Retrieved July from https://www.coneval.org.mx/Medicion/MP/Paginas/Pobreza_2016.aspx.

ConMéxico (2010). Comentarios de ConMéxico al anteproyecto denominado Lineamientos Generales para el Expendui o Distribución de Alimentos y Bebidas en los Establecimientos de Consumo Escolar de los Planteles de Educación Básica (B001002280). Comisión Nacional de Mejora Regulatoria. Communiqué ConMéxico released during the consultation process of the *Lineamientos 2010.* Available from the author on request.

Darlavuelta (n.d.). https://www.darlavuelta.com.

Diario de los Debates [*Diary of debates*], Cámara de Diputados LX Legislatura (2007) (Año I, Segundo Periodo, 10 de abril de 2007). http://cronica.diputados.gob.mx/PDF/60/2007/abr/070410-2.pdf.

Estrategia Nacional para la Prevención y el Control del Sobrepeso, la Obesidad y la Diabetes [*National Strategy for the Prevention and Control of Overweight, Obesity and Diabetes*] *(ENSOD)* (2013). Secretaría de Salud, México.

Frenk, J. (2006). Bridging the divide: Global lessons from evidence-based health policy in Mexico. *The Lancet, 368*(9539), 954–961. https://doi.org/10.1016/S0140-6736(06)69376-8.

Frenk, J., Bobadilla, J. L., Sepúlveda, J., & Cervantes, M. L. (1989). Health transition in middle-income countries: New challenges for health care. *Health Policy and Planning, 4* (1), 29–39. https://doi.org/10.1093/heapol/4.1.29.

Frenk, J., Bobadilla, J. L., Stern, C., Frejka, T., & Lozano, R. (1991). Elements for a theory of the health transition. *Health Transition Review,* 1(1), 21–38.

Frenk, J., Frejka, T., Bobadilla, J. L., Stern, C., Lozano, R., Sepúlveda, J., & José, M. (1991). La transición epidemiológica en América Latina. *Boletín de la Oficina Sanitaria Panamericana (OSP),* 111(6), 485–496. http://iris.paho.org/xmlui/handle/123456789/16560.

Gálvez, A. (2018). *Eating NAFTA: Trade, food policies, and the destruction of Mexico.* University of California Press.

Gard, M. (2010). *The end of the obesity epidemic.* Routledge.

Gard, M., & Pluim, C. (2014). *Schools and public health. Past, present and future.* Lexington Books.

Gard, M., & Wright, J. (2005). *Obesity epidemic: Science, morality and ideology.* Routledge.

Gómez, E. J. (2019). Coca-Cola's political and policy influence in Mexico: Understanding the role of institutions, interests and divided society. *Health Policy and Planning*, 34(7), 520–528. https://doi.org/10.1093/heapol/czz063.

Greenhalgh, S. (2016). Neoliberal science, Chinese style: Making and managing the 'obesity epidemic'. *Social Studies of Science*, 46(4), 485–510. https://doi.org/10.1177/0306312716655501.

Greenhalgh, S. (2019). Making China safe for Coke: How Coca-Cola shaped obesity science and policy in China. *BMJ (Clinical research ed.)*, 364, k5050. https://doi.org/10.1136/bmj.k505c.

Greenhalgh, S. (2021). Inside ILSI: How Coca-Cola, working through its scientific nonprofit, created a global science of exercise for obesity and got it embedded in Chinese policy (1995–2015). *Journal of Health Politics, Policy and Law*, 46(2), 235–276. https://doi.org/10.1215/03616878-8802174.

Guthman, J. (2011). *Weighing in: Obesity, food justice and the limits of capitalism.* University of California Press.

INEGI (2018). *Encuesta Nacional de Ingresos y Gastos de los Hogares (ENIGH)* [*National Survey of Income and Expenditure*]. https://www.inegi.org.mx/contenidos/programas/enigh/nc/2018/doc/enigh2018_ns_presentacion_resultados.pdf.

Kamat, S. (2004). The privatization of public interest: Theorizing NGO discourse in a neoliberal era. *Review of International Political Economy*, 11(1), 155–176. https://doi.org/10.1080/0969229042000179794.

Larreguy, H., Montiel Olea, C. E., & Querubin, P. (2017). Political brokers: Partisans or agents? Evidence from the Mexican Teachers' Union. *American Journal of Political Science*, 61(4), 877–891. https://doi.org/10.1111/ajps.12322.

Levinson, B. A. (2014). Education reform sparks teacher protest in Mexico. *Phi Delta Kappan*, 95(8), 48–51. https://doi.org/10.1177/003172171409500811.

Lineamientos 2010 (Acuerdo mediante el cual se establecen los lineamientos generales para el expendio o distribución de alimentos y bebidas en los establecimientos de consumo escolar de los planteles de educación básica [General guidelines for the distribution or sales of food and drinks by retailers within basic education schools]) (2010). Diario Oficial de la Federación: Órgano del Gobierno Constitucional de los Estados Unidos Mexicanos.

Lineamientos 2014 (Acuerdo mediante el cual se establecen los lineamientos generales para el expendio y distribución de alimentos y bebidas preparados y procesados en las escuelas del Sistema Educativo Nacional [Guidelines for the sales and distribution of prepared and processed food and drinks in the Mexican national education system]) (2014). Diario Oficial de la Federación: Órgano del Gobierno Constitucional de los Estados Unidos Mexicanos.

López Aguilar, M. d. J. (2013). Una reforma "educativa" contra los maestros y el derecho a la educación [An "educational" reform against teachers and the right to education]. *El Cotidiano*, 179(May–June), 55–76.

Lougheed, T. (2006). Policy: WHO/ILSI affiliation sustained. *Environmental Health Perspectives*, 114(9), A521–A521. https://doi.org/doi:10.1289/ehp.114-a521a.

Martínez-Salgado, C., & Leal-Fernández, G. (2003). Epidemiological transition: Model or illusion? A look at the problem of health in Mexico. *Social Science & Medicine*, 57(3), 539–550. https://doi.org/10.1016/S0277-9536(02)00379-00379.

MexicanosActivos (n.d.). Queremos Mexicanos Activos [We want active Mexicans]. https://mexicanosactivos.org.

Mialon, M., Ho, M., Carriedo, A., Ruskin, G., & Crosbie, E. (2021). Beyond nutrition and physical activity: Food industry shaping of the very principles of scientific integrity. *Globalization and Health*, 17(1), 37. https://doi.org/10.1186/s12992-021-00689-1.

Mintz, S. W. (1985). *Sweetness and power: The place of sugar in modern history*. Penguin Books.

Mintz, S. W. (2013). Time, sugar, and sweetness. In C. Counihan & P. Van Esterik (eds.), *Food and culture: A reader* (3rd ed., pp. 91–106). Routledge.

Moise, N., Cifuentes, E., Orozco, E., & Willett, W. C. (2011). Limiting the consumption of sugar sweetened beverages in Mexico's obesogenic environment: A qualitative policy review and stakeholder analysis. *Journal of Public Health*, 32, 458–475. https://doi.org/10.1057/jphp.2011.39.

Monterrosa, E., Campirano, F., Tolentino, L., Frongillo, E., Hernandez, S., Kawfer-Horwitz, M., & Rivera, J. (2015). Stakeholder perspectives on national policy for regulating the school food environment in Mexico. *Health Policy and Planning*, 30(1), 28–38. https://doi.org/10.1093/heapol/czt094.

Moreno-Brid, J. C., Garry, S., & Krozer, A. (2016). Minimum wages and inequality in Mexico: A Latin American perspective. *Revista de economía mundial*, issue 43, 113–129.

MOVISA (n.d.). Quiénes somos? [Who are we?]. www.movisa.org.mx.

Navarro, V. (2007). Neoliberalism as a class ideology; Or, the political causes of the growth of inequalities. *International Journal of Health Services*, 37(1), 47–62. https://doi.org/10.2190/ap65-x154-4513-r520.

Navarro, V. (2008). Neoliberalism and its consequences: The world health situation since Alma Ata. *Global Social Policy*, 8(2), 152–155. https://doi.org/10.1177/1468018108008020203.

Nestle, M. (2015). *Soda politics: Taking on big soda (and winning)*. Oxford University Press.

OECD. (n.d.-a). Average annual hours actually worked per worker. Organisation for Economic Co-operation and Development. Retrieved August 28 from https://stats.oecd.org/Index.aspx?DataSetCode=ANHRS#.

OECD. (n.d.-b). Real minimun wages. Organisation for Economic Co-operation and Development. https://stats.oecd.org/Index.aspx?DataSetCode=ANHRS.

Ornelas, C. (2008). El SNTE, Elba Esther Gordillo y el gobierno de Calderón [The SNTE, Elba Esther Gordillo and the Calderón government]. *Revista Mexicana de Investigación Educativa*, 13(37), 445–469.

Ornelas, C. (2012). *Educación, colonización y rebeldía: La herencia del pacto Calderón-Gordillo* [*Education, colonialisation and rebellion: The legacy of the Calderón-Gordillo pact*]. Siglo XXI Editores.

Otero, G. (2018). *The neoliberal diet: Healthy profits, unhealthy people*. University of Texas Press.

PepsiCo (2006). Presentan empresas de Grupo PEPSICO programa Vive Saludable [PEPSICO enterprises launch the program Live Healthy]. Press release. http://pepsico.com.mx/live/pressrelease/Presentan-Empresas-de-Grupo-PesiCo.

Plazas, M. (2010). Juego y Comida dan salud a tu vida [Eat and Play make you healthy]. *Revista Latinoamericana de Estudios Educativos*, 40(2), 153–164.

Story, M. (1999). School-based approaches for preventing and treating obesity. *International Journal of Obesity*, 23, S43–S51.

Story, M., Nanney, M., & Schwartz, M. (2009). Schools and obesity prevention: Creating school environments and policies to promote healthy eating and physical activity. *The Milbank Quarterly*, 87(1), 71–100. https://doi.org/10.1111j.1468-0009.2009.00548.x.

Swinburn, B., Egger, G., & Raza, F. (1999). Dissecting obesogenic environments: The development and application of a framework for identifying and prioritizing environmental interventions for obesity. *Preventive Medicine*, 29(6), 563–570. https://doi.org/10.1006/pmed.1999.0585.

Tenorio, J. (2022). Encountering 'healthy' food in Mexican schools. In M. Gard, D. Powell, & J. Tenorio (eds.), *Routledge handbook of critical obesity studies* (pp. 144–153). Routledge.

Treviño Ronzón, E., & Sánchez Pacheco, G. (2014). La Implementación de los Lineamientos para Regular el Expendio de Alimentos y Bebidas en dos Escuelas Telesecundarias de Veracruz. Análisis desde la Perspectiva de los Sujetos [The implementation of the Guidelines to Regulate Food and Drinks Sales in two secondary schools in Veracruz: The perspective of the participants]. *CPU-e: Revista de Investigación Educativa* 19(July–December), 60–85.

Vallgårda, S. (2015a). English obesity policies: To govern and not to govern. *Health Policy*, 119(6), 743–748. https://doi.org/10.1016/j.healthpol.2015.02.015.

Vallgårda, S. (2015b). Governing obesity policies from England, France, Germany and Scotland. *Social Science & Medicine*, 147, 317–323. https://doi.org/10.1016/j.socscimed.2015.11.006.

Vallgårda, S. (2022). Evidence as a fig leaf: Obesity policies and institutional filters in Denmark. In M. Gard, D. Powell, & J. Tenorio (eds.), *Routledge handbook of critical obesity studies* (pp. 310–318). Routledge.

Vázquez Mota, J. (2007, September 18). Mensaje de la Secretaria de Educación Pública, Josefina Vázquez Mota, en la ceremonia de lanzamiento del Programa Vive Saludable Escuelas y la firma de convenio entre ILCE, CONADE Y PepsiCo, en el Salón Jaime Torres Bodet del Museo Nacional De Antropología, en el Bosque De Chapultepec, Ciudad De México [Message from the Secretary of Public Education, Josefina Vázquez Mota, at the launch ceremony of the Live Healthy Schools Program and the signing of the agreement between ILCE, CONADE and PepsiCo, in the Jaime Torres Bodet Room of the National Museum of Anthropology, in the Bosque De Chapultepec, Mexico City]. Secretaría de Educación Pública. http://www.sep.gob.mx/wb/sep1/sep1_VersionJVM#.WBhyTt.

Vázquez Mota, J. (2007, September 27). Mensaje de la Secretaria de Educación Pública, Josefina Vázquez Mota, al participar como testigo de honor en la firma de un convenio de colaboración entre la CONADE y Mundo Bienestar, en las instalaciones del Centro Nacional de Alto Rendimiento, Ciudad Deportiva, Distrito Federal [Message from the Secretary of Public Education, Josefina Vázquez Mota, when participating as an honorary witness in the signing of a collaboration agreement between CONADE and Mundo Bienestar, at the facilities of the National High Performance Center, Ciudad Deportiva, Federal District]. Secretaría de Educación Pública. http://www.sep.gob.mx/wb/sep1/sep1_VersionJVM270907#.W.

WHO (2000). *Obesity: Preventing and managing the global epidemic: Report of a WHO consultation*. World Health Organization. https://www.who.int/nutrition/publications/obesity/WHO_TRS_894/en/.

WHO (2004). *Global strategy on diet, physical activity and health*. World Health Organization.

4 Corporatizing Healthy Eating

In 2006, after the ENSANUT 2006 announced obesity as a problem, the Veracruz state government instructed the Secretaría de Educación de Veracruz (SEV) to develop an anti-obesity strategy. In response, a group of enthusiast education authorities within the Dirección de Educación Primaria Estatal (DEPE) at the SEV designed SUMA, an educational strategy to promote healthy eating in primary schools.[1] The DEPE's team used the vertical structure around which schools are organized and overseen to expand the program across Veracruz. Even though it was designed and run without any budget attached, SUMA was implemented in schools. The program, according to its leader Victoria (see Chapter 1), was well received by teachers because it was aligned with the official curriculum and required minimal reporting.[2]

In 2010, after Nestlé and the DEPE started a partnership to promote healthy lifestyles in schools across the state, SUMA was changed. That same year, Nestlé had started the implementation of its program Nutrir, the Mexican version of its global Nestlé Healthy Kids program, in one school in central Veracruz.[3] Nutrir was part of Nestlé's Creating Shared Value (CSV), which seeks to "empower" people across Nestlé's value chain so that value is created for anyone as much as for Nestlé. Veracruz is rich in coffee, sugar and milk. Nestlé has strong interests in and benefits from what this area offers. Their form of "giving back" to the community is to provide children with information on how to be 'healthy'. In 2010, SUMA and Nutrir became one program: SUMA-Nutrir; partly funded and guided by Nestlé and partly guided and completely operationalized by Victoria and her team.[4]

Based on the notion that 'fighting' obesity is a shared responsibility between the public and private sectors (Chapter 3), corporations have launched myriad health-promotion programs—operated by their philanthropy departments—and partnered with state agencies for implementation. These partnerships are problematic due to the ambivalence between corporate interests and public health goals. There is considerable research into how public–private (or public–corporate, as I prefer to call them) partnerships in public health have been discursively articulated (Herrick, 2009; Ruckert & Labonté, 2014; Vander Schee & Boyles, 2010). Yet how these partnerships have been actually enacted, and with what effects, remains largely unexplored.[5]

DOI: 10.4324/9781003356264-4

The discussion around SUMA-Nutrir and its effects presented in this chapter addresses this gap. This chapter shows how "shared responsibility" operates in the day-to-day and the issues that arise from a partnership with two unequal partners. The DEPE-Nestlé collaboration was beneficial for both parties in various ways. Poorly resourced, lacking funding and within a bureaucratic system, DEPE staff found in Nestlé what they required to grow their health-promotion initiative. Nestlé offered its management capability, but most importantly it provided the economic resource that never came from the state. In exchange, Nestlé gained the expertise and in-depth contextual knowledge of Victoria and her experienced team, and their committed labor, for free. Through this partnership, Nestlé expanded its presence and interests across Veracruz.

Herrick (2009, p. 55) criticizes corporate social responsibility (CSR) health-promotion programs because they employ a health rhetoric that "constructs choice and information as a form of consumer empowerment". Citing a variety of actions carried out by Unilever, PepsiCo, Coca-Cola and Nestlé under the umbrella of CSR, Herrick concludes that CSR, when underpinned by the personal choice argument, shifts the blame for health outcomes from the industry to individuals. Building on this literature, in this chapter I show that the SEV–Nestlé partnerships triggered by the shared responsibility discourse have had effects other than simply making 'healthy' Mexicans. As I demonstrate through the case of SUMA-Nutrir, these partnerships have aided the construction of a corporate project that seeks to govern one of the most basic biological functions: eating.

The regulation of the biological functions of human beings, what Foucault (2007, 2008) calls bio-politics, has, since the nineteenth century, become a political strategy through which the individual and social body has been governed. In Mexico, as Chapter 2 showed, education campaigns in the early twentieth century aimed to change the eating and hygiene practices of the population to make them 'modern'. However, the way in which bodies are administered and the management of life is calculated has changed. Neoliberal bio-politics, Foucault (2008, p. 242) argues, seeks to extend an "enterprise form"; that is, the economic model of "supply and demand and of investment-costs-profit so as to make it a model of social relations and of existence itself, a form of relationship of the individual to himself, time, those around him, the group, and the family". As a tool aimed to control the social and individual body through 'healthy' eating, SUMA-Nutrir is part of what I refer to as a "corporate bio-political project".

In this chapter, I draw on interviews with education authorities at the SEV and with a Nestlé representative, Claudia, and on observations conducted across the meetings and schools visits they invited me to "follow". Interrogating the workings and politics of SUMA-Nutrir, I show how the *dispositif of healthy lifestyles* has enabled corporations to use public resources, like human resources from the SEV, to articulate and disseminate a sophisticated project that uses school food practices as a vehicle to expand their influence among Mexicans. As a public–corporate partnership, I suggest, SUMA-Nutrir epitomizes the extent to which neoliberalism is configuring cultural practices and advancing corporate interests at the same time.

In what follows, I explain how the shared responsibility discourse enabled Nestlé to co-opt the DEPE's health work. Also, I demonstrate how, through a perspective on 'health' that is tied to rationales of self-government and choice, Nestlé has articulated a complex project that draws on the *saludable* language and on the construction of numbers to govern the health of Mexicans. Some readers might consider that I am depicting Nestlé as a homogenous entity and that I have deployed a top-down analysis.[6] My ultimate aim, however, is not to vilify Nestlé, but to show what happens when state employees are pushed to rely on corporate resources due to the inaction of the Mexican state to provide aid to its population.

The Corporate Government of Eating

On a foggy morning in late May 2016, I accompanied Victoria to a primary school in Xalapa, Veracruz state's capital, where she would chat with the four women who sold food during the break. The visit was part of Victoria's usual supervision routine to oversee the implementation of the *Lineamientos* and SUMA-Nutrir. Victoria initiated the conversation with the women describing the "pervasiveness" of obesity in Mexico and in the school. "According to the results of our survey, this school is the second place in obesity amongst primary schools in the state", she asserted. Using data collected through SUMA-Nutrir, she made the problem clear to the women, "according to the FIA,[7] there are 24 cases of obesity here". Referencing the *Lineamientos* and SUMA-Nutrir, Victoria encouraged the women to reduce fats and sugars in their cooking, and to limit the food options and portions served.

"I used to sell *esquites* with all the toppings. However",[8] one of the women said proudly, "I'm avoiding mayonnaise as you suggested. Kids are still buying them because there's no other option". "Exactly! We have to limit the options and substitute products. Some products are better than others. I'm brand-free, so I can tell you which of them are better", Victoria answered, assuring the women that she would provide a list of products to be avoided. At the end of the chat, the principal highlighted the school's commitment to promoting "healthier diets" and described the constraints to achieve this goal. "Junk food" consumption had been halted in the school. Nonetheless, students brought these "unhealthy products" from the outside. "Prohibition is never enough", Victoria remarked, "that's why it is better to teach the kids to make informed choices".

The interactions between Victoria and the four women evidenced how discourse spread Nestlé's notions of health and food, trying to inscribe them into cooking practices. As we walked away from the classroom where the meeting had been held, one of the four women approached Victoria to ask whether she could keep selling *tamales* in the break time. Influenced by the language used by Victoria, the woman started the conversation emphasizing the nutritional quality of her *tamales*. "I make them healthy [*sanos*]. I don't use lard or other fats, only *masa*, chicken and chili".

Victoria congratulated the woman, but also emphasized that more effort needed to be put into changing students' eating practices. Victoria concluded the conversation encouraging the four cooks to consider the students like their own children. "Many students", Victoria emphasized, "have their first meal here at the school, so if we take care of our children at home, we have to take care of the students' nutrition here in the school". Victoria's perspective on the relationship between food, maternal responsibility and obesity was clearly framed by the discourses within the *dispositif of healthy lifestyles*. While Victoria spoke about caring through food, as others did during my fieldwork, she considered, imbued by the *dispositif*, the provision of "good" and "healthy" food as a moral question. For her, mothers, both at home and at schools, have to provide food "responsibly" to avoid children becoming fat.

SUMA-Nutrir has worked as a tool to manage and discipline the population through education, surveillance and the production of reports, surveys and visual materials. The above story shows how this program has channeled healthy lifestyles into discursive practices in schools. Victoria entered this school as a public servant. Nevertheless, she was also spreading Nestlé's ideas about food and its relationship to health. Her message was aligned with the message that corporations and pro-market reformers have deployed through healthy lifestyles: a good state of health is ultimately a matter of personal responsibility that can be attained through making good choices.

SUMA-Nutrir's actions moralized mothers and endowed them with the responsibility of providing 'healthy foods', regulating portions and forging nutritionally informed children. According to Rose (2001), neoliberal bio-politics seek to create "active" partners that accept their "responsibility" in securing their own wellbeing. Nestlé's CSV strategies have succeeded in making Mexicans, especially mothers, interiorize the "enterprise form" that is vital for the success of neoliberalism.

Victoria, a mother herself, interiorized the enterprise form in her own construction as a mother: "Now that I have more information, I have achieved changes in my household. I thought I was good at cooking, but I'm not. Now that I have other ideas, I've improved. I can see changes in my family". Victoria spoke from two standpoints: as a program coordinator and as a mother. These perspectives mingled and enabled her to bring family affairs into her health work and vice versa. Victoria painted herself as the desirable final construction of the good mother: someone who looks for nutrition and health information, appropriates it and applies it responsibly in the day-to-day care of the household. This can be observed when Victoria told me how the nutritional information that she learned through SUMA-Nutrir helped her to offer 'healthier' food to her family. "Before", she exclaimed, "I thought that cooking lentils was good. I used to say, today I've prepared a very good meal for my family, I did it well. However, I cooked lentils with chorizo, bacon and ham, because I was taught that way".

I am not going to discuss whether the change of ingredients in cooking lentils is good or not. What is important to highlight is how corporate bio-politics permeated the construction of the good mother. In the context of abundant 'unhealthy' foods, mothers have to educate themselves to take informed decisions based more on calories and nutrition than flavor and tradition. Making mothers think of food in terms of calories and portions is key for the bio-political control of the population. "When I cooked lentils with plantain [instead of the other ingredients]", Victoria said, highlighting the positive results of the SUMA-Nutrir activities and what she had learned, "my family enjoyed them and I said, 'Wow, I've cut the number of calories significantly', and I realized that I did not cook well, though I believed I did!".

The family, as a singular social group, and mothers, as individuals, are the "target groups" of Nestlé's bio-political project. But why the family and mothers? Neoliberal bio-politics, Foucault claims, extends the enterprise form in the management of life. Market forms of organization, like detailed planning, evaluation of outcomes and a cost–profit logic, are imposed over the control of social relationships, Foucault (2008, pp. 243–244) explains, like the mother–daughter one:

> the mother-children relationship, concretely characterized by the time spent by the mother with the child, the quality of the care she gives, the affection she shows, the vigilance with which she follows its development, its education, and not only its scholastic but also its physical progress, the way in which she not only gives it food but also imparts a particular style to eating patterns, and the relationship she has with its eating, all constitute for the neo-liberals an investment which can be measured in time.

The *dispositif of healthy lifestyles* has depicted the good, responsible mother as someone who is literate in health and nutrition and uses this knowledge to make family members, especially children, conscious about the need of eating 'healthily'.[9] The investment of time and resources to manage vital functions, such as eating and moving, will be traduced, in the long term, into what corporate bio-politics depicts as a responsible-good citizen. In exchange, corporations will profit from this good individual/responsible consumer who is able to make 'healthy' and 'informed' choices.

SUMA-Nutrir enabled Nestlé to advance its bio-political project. The multiple activities comprised in this program deployed moralizing discourses that made individuals responsible for their own health failures. In the name of achieving good health, therefore, food needs to be considered in terms of its biological nature and its caloric content. This claim is neatly represented in the words of Claudia, a member of Nestlé's Creating Shared Value Department in Mexico.[10] I chatted with Claudia to know more about the workings and politics of Nutrir. In a rather articulated way, Claudia explained to me Nestlé's philanthropic philosophy and the variety of actions to improve nutrition the company made. The aim of Nestlé's 'healthy' eating programs, she stated, was to change food culture in schools and beyond:

> We are going to change four habits: feed your child according to their age, measure your portions, choose nutritional foods and get active daily [...] Portions is another topic that we haven't paid attention to. At Nestlé we see that as a need, because in the Mexican culture food is love. So, the more you

eat, the more you are showing love to others. It is quite common that you can't leave the dining table until you have finished the portion in your plate. And also, it is common that grannies ask, 'Do you want another serving in your plate, my son?' 'Yes, granny, I love you, give me more' [¿Otro platito, mijo? Pues sí abuelita, te quiero, dame otro.]. And that's wrong! That's something very warm in our culture, it's quite kind and makes us different to other countries, but we have to change it!

Informing people, particularly mothers, of the need to become aware of measuring the quantity and frequency of food was at the heart of the SEV–Nestlé partnership. Serving more food than what an individual should consume based on nutritional formulas was seen as a cultural weakness that Nestlé had to change. Candid generosity cannot remain attached to food. Instead, according to Claudia, Victoria and other people that I interviewed, mothers need to be more educated in nutrition to provide only the required calories and never excessive food.

Yet obviously this project of government was not arbitrarily imposed in a top-down way. The content of SUMA-Nutrir was produced and negotiated among the partners involved in the program. The DEPE staff was also aware of the politics behind the healthy eating messages that Nestlé was trying to push through some materials. An example in this regard was explained to me by Mario, Victoria's manager within the DEPE. In 2016, the SUMA-Nutrir team at the DEPE produced a poster listing ten actions children should follow to be healthy. All the recommendations were aimed at maintaining the energy balance. The DEPE team consulted the content of this poster with Claudia. According to Mario, none of the listed actions were controversial except for the last one, which said: "Stop! Resist temptation and eat until you're at home".[11] "Claudia didn't agree with the point in the poster that says: 'Stop!'", Mario emphasized, explaining that he had openly problematized that this message was not good for Nestlé, but that it was important.

Transforming SUMA into SUMA-Nutrir represented benefits for all parties. Both Nestlé and the DEPE used their resources and expertise—although only partially and subject to debate—to reach their goals in promoting healthy lifestyles. The DEPE staff's deep knowledge of the education system and local politics was vital for the success of SUMA-Nutrir in Veracruz. Nestlé's vast economic resources and skills in entrepreneurial management facilitated the production of printed materials like cookbooks and posters, the dissemination of the program across the state and close supervision of the program roll-out by its creators.

However, without denying the agency of the DEPE staff, there were occasions when Nestlé's interests prevailed over those of the public. Nestlé used SUMA-Nutrir, and the labor of public servants, to disseminate its perspectives on health, food and nutrition among teachers, parents and students. Unlike in other Mexican states, where Nestlé was not lucky enough to find a "committed team from the government", as Claudia said, in Veracruz it discovered a team of education authorities deeply devoted to health work and with an ongoing, locally created strategy that was already showing results. Without undermining Nestlé's good philanthropic intentions, it can be said that its program achieved its goals of impact by piggybacking on SUMA's extended work. The group of committed education advisers at the DEPE untaintedly aided the corporate bio-political project.

Nestlé has been actively implementing CSV strategies related to nutrition education and health promotion around the world through the program Nestlé Healthy Kids, recently rebranded as Nestlé for Healthier Kids (N4HK).[12] Nestlé's CSV initiatives are outlined by its headquarters in Switzerland then exported globally for implementation with the aid of "partners", either NGOs or state agencies. Countries where Nestlé operates, both from the First or the Third Worlds, are targeted, but more emphasis is put on countries which produce raw materials. Scholars from different fields have critically reviewed the CSV idea, exposing its deficiencies and double intentionality. Crane et al. (2014), for instance, have argued that CSV is problematic because it overlooks the "tensions" between social and economic goals. Shamir (2004) points out that private industry creates CSR and CSV projects to increase its market competitiveness and to improve its corporate image. Leone et al. (2015) consider that, through CSR programs, some corporations are shifting the message from "eat less" to "move more", thus attributing greater responsibility to consumers. This is true in Mexico.

Nestlé conceives that having a 'healthy' population is a requirement for its own business expansion and sustainability. This can be seen in Nestlé's 2014 *Creating Shared Value Report*, where it argues why "promoting healthy lifestyles" is important for the corporation: "we have always believed that over the long term, healthy populations, healthy economies and healthy business performance are mutually reinforcing" (Nestlé, 2015, p. 49). Nestlé's strategies seek to control the health and lives of people around the world to expand its markets and maintain its businesses performance. Schools are invaluable spaces for this project.

Making Cookbooks *Saludables*

In the second week of April 2016, I attended a meeting in Xalapa between SEV authorities, Claudia from Nestlé and a group of chefs. The meeting was to discuss Nutrir's expansion across the SEV and to select the recipes that would form the second volume of a "regional cookbook". When I arrived at the meeting room in the SEV building, Victoria and others were already there. Claudia arrived a few minutes later and looked surprised when she saw I was there. "What are you doing here?", she exclaimed. The meeting started by 10 am. In the first hour, Pablo, the Director of External Engagement at the SEV, and Claudia talked about two key changes coming up in the SEV–Nestlé collaboration. After four years of joint implementation across the schools managed by the DEPE, SUMA-Nutrir would split at the beginning of the 2016–2017 school year. SUMA would remain working within the DEPE and Nutrir alone would expand to high schools across Veracruz, managed by other directorates within the SEV.

Another change in the SEV–Nestlé partnership would involve funding. From 2012 to 2016, under SUMA-Nutrir, printed materials and other resources had been distributed across primary schools to aid teachers' health-promotion work. Most were produced by Victoria and her team, but Nestlé had absorbed the printing costs. Also, as DEPE staff told me, Nestlé covered some travel and event expenses. However, since Nutrir would soon grow exponentially, doubling the number of schools already included, a new implementation scheme was required. Nestlé's desire to expand its program matched its desire to minimize costs, and technology offered a solution. Nestlé would digitize all materials and developed a website where teachers could access Nutrir and download the resources. DEPE staff would instruct their peers in the use of the platform.

One of the materials that would be digitized was the cookbook *Comiendo bien a lo Veracruz-sano* [Eating Well in Healthy-Veracruz-style] (Nestlé México, 2013). The English translation, "Eating Well in a Healthy-Veracruz-style", does not capture the complexity implied in the title. "Veracruz-sano" is a play on the word "veracruzano", which is the noun and adjective identifying people from the state of Veracruz. Boldly, the cookbook editors played with words to assign a positive nutritional value to the recipes included. *Veracruz-sano*, then, refers to a cooking style native to the state of Veracruz that is also good for people's health.

This cookbook includes recipes using "regional ingredients" to "teach mothers" that cooking 'healthy' is not expensive, as Victoria described it to me. *Comiendo bien a lo Veracruz-sano* was the result of a contest for "local recipes", where mothers from across the state submitted their recipes. Victoria, her colleagues and people from Nestlé selected the "most representative" and "healthy" recipes that included "traditional ingredients". Four thousand copies were printed, using Nestlé funding, and then distributed by the DEPE. Victoria and her colleagues had significant control over the production of the cookbook. In 2012, when it was produced, the DEPE and Nestlé partnership was still maturing. Yet things changed as both sides committed more time, expertise and resources to promote 'healthy' eating in Veracruz.

In the second hour of the meeting, SEV authorities, Victoria and her team, Claudia from Nestlé and three local chefs selected the recipes that would form the *Comiendo Bien a lo Veracruz-sano* volume II (Nestlé México, 2016). To this end, more than 200 recipes were displayed one-by-one on the projector. The chefs and Victoria reviewed each recipe against three criteria. First, the selection of recipes was based on their "originality". Second, they should include a "regional" ingredient from Veracruz. Finally, recipes were selected based on how 'healthy' they were.

Diverse knowledges and interests competed in determining whether a recipe was original and healthy or not. The chefs' judgement came from two middle-class men who were from a civil-society organization that sought to strengthen the relationships among the restaurant and food-industry sectors. Victoria, for her part, expressed her opinion as a mother, as a teacher and as an education authority who had to balance the selection of recipes from across the state's multiple school districts. Originality was trivial in some cases. While some recipes contained a clearly identifiable local ingredient, in other recipes ingredient names had been changed to use Veracruz terminology to make them "local". Claudia barely expressed an opinion. She was carefully paying attention to the exchange of ideas. She only intervened once when Victoria and the chefs disagreed about the 'nutritious' quality of the food made through a particular recipe. "Let's include a healthy option [*opción saludable*] for each recipe", Claudia stated firmly in this case.

Changes like a stronger emphasis on the word *saludable*, the incorporation of explicit messages promoting a 'healthy' diet and a more frequent display of Nestlé's logos are included in the 2016 edition of the cookbook. In the 2013 version of *Comiendo Bien a lo Veracruz-sano*, the word *saludable* was used only twice, but in the second volume *saludable* appears in nearly 100 recipes. The number of times *saludable* is used across both cookbooks is relevant because Nestlé had a deeper in-put into the second cookbook and shows the extent to which corporate forces gained the right to frame what is 'healthy'. Before Nestlé expanded the *saludable* discourse in SUMA, the DEPE staff who created the program used only the words *sano/sana*. This is evident in the materials produced before the partnership with Nestlé, and it is also clear how *saludable* gained more terrain as the collaboration progressed.

Following Claudia's advice during the meeting, a "healthy" [*saludable*] option was included for each of the 97 recipes in the *Comiendo Bien a lo Veracruz-sano* volume II. To make a dish 'healthy', for example, recipes direct cooks to swap lard for oil, grill foods instead of frying them, avoid added sugar and to limit portion sizes. Messages encouraging people from Veracruz to eat well and have a 'healthy' life do not appear only in the recipes. The phrase "No hay alimentos buenos ni malos, solo mide las porciones de los alimentos accesorios" [Food is neither good nor bad, only be aware of the portions of accessory foods] is located at the beginning of the desserts section. Interestingly, this message is followed by a coconut treat recipe whose ingredients are "shredded fresh coconut" and "one large can of condensed milk". The 'healthy' option of this recipe is "to consume only one portion a day and avoid frequent consumption" (Nestlé México, 2016, pp. 84–85).

This is an implicit reference to one of Nestlé's most famous products in Mexico, the condensed milk called "La Lechera". This product's brand name is widely used to refer to condensed milk in general, and its inclusion is an example of how Nestlé is positioned in the new cookbook and uses it to sneakily promote its own products.

Creating and using cookbooks as a mechanism to reach a broader audience is not new for Nestlé. As Aguilar-Rodríguez (2009) has documented through her analysis of cookbooks in twentieth-century Mexico, Nestlé relied heavily on cookbooks to expand its emerging market in Mexico in the 1950s and 1960s. In those cookbooks, of course, the 'nutritional' quality of the recipes was not highlighted, because that discourse was not useful then. Instead, cookbooks drew on the modernity discourse as their vehicle to attract the enlarging middle-classes which emerged during the "Mexican Miracle".

Today, Nestlé's cookbooks portray the corporation's 'efforts' to make 'healthier' people in Veracruz. For this purpose, pictures showing Nutrir materials and cheery students wearing chef's hats and aprons bearing Nestlé's logo appear throughout the cookbooks. With these recent cookbooks, Nestlé used recipes, ingredients and cooking practices to unite the state of Veracruz under the label of 'healthy'. However, the two volumes of the cookbook did not look exclusively to disseminate 'traditional' ingredients and recipes. Instead, they created space for Nestlé to keep expanding its business interests in the state. But, as I mentioned in the introduction to this chapter, the use of the *saludable* language was only one of the tools that Nestlé employed to disseminate its perspectives on health. The other one was the construction and uses of numbers, as I elaborate in what follows.

The Construction and Uses of Numbers

During our interview at her office in Nestlé's headquarters in Mexico City in April 2016, Claudia always had a computer with her. She used it to show me graphics, tables and statistics when answering my questions about the evolution of Nutrir across Mexico. One graphic displayed a timeline with the number of schools and students reached by the program from 2006 to 2015 in two states: Veracruz and the State of Mexico.[13] "The State of Mexico and Veracruz are the two states in the country with the greatest number of public primary schools and where there is also an issue of obesity and of malnutrition", Claudia stated, adding that those were some of the criteria why Nestlé had chosen those states to implement Nutrir. Yet another important reason why Nestlé's CSV strategy was deployed in these places was because of their strategic nature for them. Victoria knew this. "I know that Nestlé picked us [the state of Veracruz] because they have factories here, and that is one of the reasons why they select states [to implement their CSV strategies]", she declared.

One of the main differences between SUMA alone and SUMA-Nutrir was that the latter barely required reporting from teachers. This changed when Nestlé partnered with the DEPE to promote healthy eating in Veracruz. The recording and collection of evidence (photographs and reports) became crucial to the workings of SUMA-Nutrir. Teachers started to collect data from students with regards their eating and living practices and to report on the implementation of the program. Each school collected these data to report them to the DEPE. The impact of Nestlé's Nutrir was assessed against the number of students, parents and teachers who were reported as engaged with it. Numbers also represented vital data from the thousands of peoples involved with the program.[14] Numbers, and the narratives around their creation and use, captured my attention due to their centrality in supporting the need for and the relevance of public–corporate partnerships like SUMA-Nutrir. In what follows, I show that the narratives around the construction of numbers through SUMA-Nutrir—data about individuals, the number of schools covered, the number of 'trained' teachers, and so on—shed light on the ongoing corporatization of health. My intention is to bring the reader's attention to the complex politics behind the construction of those numbers.

Nestlé started to run Nutrir in the State of Mexico in 2009, just as the expansion of one of its most important coffee factories began there.[15] However, the program was not as successful as it was in Veracruz. "The biggest challenge", Claudia asserted when I asked why, "has been to find a team from the government devoted to implementing the program, it is very hard for us, as a private business, to operate the program. So, what we really need is commitment". "Veracruz is a great, successful case", Claudia emphasized, "because that team *really have* owned the program". Numbers made success tangible. "We started with 450,000 kids in Veracruz. From this year", Claudia said pointing to section of the timeline in the 2012 segment, where a steady growth in 'impact' could be seen, "you can see that luckily in Veracruz we have added new students to the program each school year, and we've been doing so until today".

The materials that Claudia let me observe on her screen reflected the number of schools that had been part of the program and the number of students, teachers and parents who had been "taught". Those numbers were important because, in a simple visual way, they expressed the material representation of how many people were "adopting" a 'healthy lifestyle'. Those numbers supported the argument that Nestlé's CSV strategies were having a highly positive impact on making 'healthier' people. Impact was measured by counting the number of teachers, students and parents 'trained' by Nutrir alone and by SUMA-Nutrir through schools. The growing participation of schools represented in numbers was used by Nestlé to demonstrate the success of its program.

The material representation of healthy lifestyles in numbers is quite important for corporate bio-politics. Reaching more schools, 'training' more teachers and 'educating' more mothers is the ultimate aim of a system of government that has accountability and profitability at its heart. Promoting healthy lifestyles across schools and families might not be increasing the sales of Nestlé products, but, as the data of this research make evident, it is undeniably making the brand more present in these social spaces. Accountability is key to achieving profitability. The greater the impact that is reported, the better valued a program will be. In the desire for a greater impact, 'health' is to some extent reduced to the number of schools and families that have been part of a program.

The 'impact' of Nestlé's healthy lifestyles programs, grouped under their global strategy United for Healthier Kids (U4HK), also has been validated by researchers. Drewnowski et al. (2018), for instance, highlight the success of the Mexican U4HK experience, encouraging other corporations to adopt this "novel" and successful public–private partnership as a guide. In this paper, the authors, who are either Nestlé employees or members of the U4HK advisory board, described how the different programs targeting families and children through diverse spaces is making them "healthier". Facebook, YouTube and Twitter campaigns are reported to have reached a total of "13.5 million exposures to the audience in 2014". An additional "34 million exposures of the U4HK messages" were also generated "in the form of published articles, mass media releases, and blogs". In more connection to schools, this paper reports that "40 000 Eatwell Plates", "designed to help families balance the intake of different food groups", were distributed to parents and students "to provide information about portion size" (pp. 813–814).

When DEPE staff worked only with SUMA, as described above, the data generated were minimal. These data remained for internal DEPE use. Things changed when the public–corporate venture SUMA-Nutrir started. Height and weight measures, health reports, socio-economic status and a full range of details from primary-school students were captured in electronic platforms. What children had for breakfast, lunch and dinner was recorded. Pictures and videos of various SUMA-Nutrir activities were produced. In the name of 'fighting' obesity, Nestlé accessed these data and used them for its own purposes.

The activities carried out under SUMA-Nutrir, mentioned across this chapter, contributed to the numbers demonstrating impact. The schools I visited with Victoria and the schools where nutrition workshops took place are surely part of the "5,000 primary schools" in Veracruz that Nestlé México reports as having impacted (Nestlé México, 2015). Also, Nestlé's (2019, p. 17) *Creating Shared Value* report states that the number of students in these schools comprise the "29 million children reached by [the] Nestlé for Healthier Kids program globally". Corporate bio-politics reduces health to numbers; numbers that validate corporate interventions and that govern the population through reducing food to portion sizes and quantifiable calories. Thus, in corporate bio-politics, numbers work for business profits as they work for public health.

Under corporate bio-politics, numbers became valuable data that can be exploited for the benefit of corporations. During my interview with Pablo, the Director of External Engagement at the SEV, he explained that Nutrir alone, as described above, would expand without SUMA to other Directorates within the SEV. Accordingly, Nutrir would become an online-only program. When I asked Pablo about Nutrir's future within the SEV, he mentioned something that supports my point:

> We hope that a large number of schools register on the platform [Nutrir's website]. Nestlé will follow this up and then they will give us the statistics and the results that they have collected from the schools working with the interactive platform.

Not only corporations have benefited from the numbers generated through health-promotion programs. While perhaps Nestlé, due to its greater resources and managerial skills, has more obviously collected numbers and used them for its own purpose, public institutions and public servants have also made use of them. Victoria provided an interesting example of this:

> Right now, we also have the Ficha Individual Acumulativa [FIA] that is the students' online health record. Some examples of the data that we have about the students are height, weight, BMI, and the noncommunicable diseases like overweight, obesity and malnutrition. So, when other institutions discovered that we have this database of almost 400,000 students, all of them, of course, wanted the database to direct their own programs.

Victoria was narrating how a recently created Consejo Estatal de Alimentación Saludable y Actividad Física para la Lucha Contra el Sobrepeso y la Obesidad en Veracruz (Consejo, for short) [Council to Fight Overweight and Obesity through Healthy Diet and Physical Activity in the State of Veracruz] worked, and what her role and experiences in it had been. The Consejo united the health, education, natural resources and social welfare secretariats of the Veracruz government. Its purpose was to coordinate actions between them to tackle obesity in Veracruz. Victoria was sent to Consejo meetings by her superiors to represent the SEV. The numbers that SUMA-Nutrir generated, and that Victoria and her team collected, were very valuable for policy design and implementation in other state-level departments. "I can tell you where the most undernourished children are", Victoria said, as she described how she had helped the DIF [the national family welfare agency],[16] the state government's welfare department, direct its school breakfast program.

Analyzing the work on poverty by an alliance of three NGOs in Mumbai, Appadurai (2001) shows that the effectiveness of this alliance in political negotiations lay in its capacity to generate and control data about a large number of families and households. Thus, Appadurai (2001, p. 34) writes, the alliance is "keenly aware of the power that this kind of knowledge—and ability—gives it". In a similar way, Victoria was keenly aware of the power that having a database of "almost 400,000 students" represented for her, and she consequently used it to expand the health work that she and her colleagues were doing:

> Just recently, people from the DIF at the federal level came here. They are creating a country-wide weight and height record. So, they are asking each state, in our case through the SEV, to create those records. I told them, 'Well, I have the FIA and I have this record of 400,000 students... not only from this year, but from the last 3 years. Is it useful for you?'

The number of schools 'trained', the reports of the kinds and quantities of food eaten by students each day, families' socioeconomic conditions and vital health-related details about students constitute precious data for any organization interested in promoting healthy lifestyles. These data were considered solid evidence of the state of students' health in Veracruz and were used to justify the need for corporate intervention. Yet this evidence reduces health to a mere numerical expression that rules out the complex cultural, political and economic processes that accompany the construction of numbers. As Escobar (2011) suggests, these numbers should instead be analyzed in "terms of ... [their] political consequences, the way in which ... [they reflect] the crafting of subjectivities, the shaping of culture, and the construction of social power" (p. 213).

An excessive emphasis on the value of the numbers made Victoria miss one important point: these data had been generated by teachers, principals and the educational authorities themselves. In Chapter 1, I told a personal story of my experience as an education adviser 'collecting' data for the public–corporate program Ponte al 100, a partnership between Coca-Cola and the Mexican government. I mentioned that amidst limited resources and time pressure, my more experienced colleagues encouraged me to "invent numbers" and upload them to the online platform before the official deadline. In my fieldwork, I observed a similar case at Benito Juárez Primary School. At around 2 pm on a hot May day in 2016, I was in the principal's office. As usual, teachers were coming in to sign on to their shift before heading to their classroom. Two male teachers, Pedro and Luis, came in laughing and greeted me. They were talking about uploading the students' marks online when Pedro asked Luis if he had already gotten the weight and height of his students. Luis, surprised, was silent for a few minutes, then replied that he did not know about that requirement. "Is this because of you, José?", Luis asked me jokingly. He then suggested that it might have been because of my research and my presence in the school that the SEV required those data. The deadline to upload the information was the following day. "I have not done it, have you?", Luis said. "Neither have I", Pedro replied, and continued, "but don't worry, let's just invent the measurements. It is all about paperwork and time-consuming stuff". Both teachers laughed loudly, said goodbye and left the room.

These stories show that numbers, while undeniably material, are produced within human interactions. Yet when considered as 'hard' data that are used to represent the usefulness of health-promotion programs and the extent to which people are, or are not, 'healthy', numbers are always produced within the complex context of people's day-to-day lives. Therefore, thinking that a school has many "cases of obesity", as Victoria expressed during the school visit, or that thousands of schools are 'healthier' just because numbers show it, might not be as accurate as many people think. Social reality is much more complex than that. A detailed exploration of the micropolitics of food and its practices in schools might help people, and policymakers, see the insignificance of what are believed to be 'good' obesity solutions: that is what I have tried to capture in Chapters 5 and 6. But before this, I discuss how the bio-political project of corporations has been enabled, not just by the effects of neoliberalism, but also by the inaction of the Mexican state to give aid to its population.

Conclusion

By the end of my interview with Claudia, she stressed that Nestlé is the company that allocates more funding for "research in nutrition in the entire world". To leave no doubt about her claim, Claudia described to me another nutrition-related project that Nestlé México had funded and developed, this time "hand in hand" with a national health institute. "We conducted a survey using a similar methodology to that of ENSANUT, but with some design modifications to obtain more data about what Mexicans eat in one day, at what time and, even, what they are doing while eating". The results of this research, sponsored by Nestlé via its Fondo Nestlé para la Nutrición [Nestlé's Nutrition Research Fellowships] that is managed by FUNSALUD, were published in the book *Qué y cómo comemos los Mexicanos* [*What and how Mexicans eat*] (Arvizú Martínez, Polo Oteyza, & Shamah Levy, 2015).

According to Claudia, public–private partnerships were Nestlé's quintessential mechanism to promote healthy lifestyles, both at the policymaking and implementation levels. Claudia, however, also acknowledged that public–private partnerships generate much debate: "why the private sector! What are you giving to them? Corporations are not paying taxes!". Therefore, "transparent" agreements between state and non-state actors needed to be established to generate trust in public–private partnerships. To highlight Nestlé's will to collaborate with the public sector towards a "shared goal", Claudia mentioned that 'United for Healthier Kids' had been launched at the Secretaría de Salud in Mexico City, after receiving the endorsement of secretary of health Mercedes Juan. "If we all collaborate around the same goal", Claudia underlined, "we can do more".

Claudia depicted Nestlé as a much-needed enterprise for Mexico. Not only did it contribute to having a healthy population, but Nestlé also contributed to the broader "progress" of Mexico.

Claudia's discourse is part of a larger narrative that presents corporations as charitable entities that create jobs, strengthen communities and care for individuals and the environment as they profit. This narrative is not necessarily new. Yet it has been further intensified as global trade liberalization and economic deregulation have increased the power and profits of corporations, and therefore their capacity to shape policy. The role the state plays in the government of the population has been equally changed. Public–corporate partnerships, which are widely celebrated in the obesity policy world, have grown exponentially as the state was downsized.

These partnerships are not intrinsically bad, but they can be dangerous. Corporate interests and public health messages are equally channeled through these partnerships. Resistance against the corporate framing of eating and cooking exists within these partnerships, as this chapter has highlighted, yet the power asymmetry between the "partners" tips the balance towards the corporate side. Through the discussion of Nestlé's fruitful partnership with the DEPE in Veracruz, this chapter has shown how the shared responsibility and the energy balance discourses framed messages around food and its relation to health to serve corporate interests.

In Chapter 2, I described how Mexico has moved from being a corporatist state to a neoliberal state, and the implications of this change on the management of the population. And, as discussed in Chapter 3, the anti-obesity policy agenda embodies and is shaped by a neoliberal form of government that has favored the expansion of corporate influence over people's lives. In this chapter, I have shown how Nestlé has crafted a complex project that seeks to regulate school food practices and, overall, change culture in Mexico. In this process, carried out through its CSV program, Nestlé has also expanded its image and interests among the population. Yet a less narrow analysis would also need to explain the conditions which enabled this to happen. The reasons why the DEPE staff became more and more reliant on Nestlé's funds, for example, was facilitated by the lack of resources provided by the state. The state is usually envisaged as an established and unified entity that administers the economy, enforces the law and organizes social life. However, these tasks are not enacted by a single entity but by a multiplicity of branches, levels and personnel that act as part of or on behalf of the state (Gupta, 2012; Sharma, 2008).

Healthy lifestyles strategies in Mexico have been released either with no funding attached or with some resources that, due to rampant corruption, rarely reach their destination. In 2016, the then Governor of Veracruz (2010–2016), Javier Duarte, was prosecuted for looting public funds, which primarily had been allocated to the education and health sectors (Semple, 2017; Watson, 2016). Yet most strategies, sooner or later, are deployed in schools in some form. This speaks of the heterogeneity of the state, and of government. Victoria and her team, as public education authorities, can be considered as an extension of the state: their practices contributed to the everyday making of the state and thereby to the project of governing the health of the population. Also, while in essence they are public servants, the DEPE staff also aided the expansion of Nestlé's bio-political project.

The staff behind SUMA were committed state workers who lacked resources, so Nestlé took up the role of funder. DEPE staff designed health-promotion materials and courses and tested them. After negotiations on how to meet the goals and perspectives of both Nestlé and the DEP, the materials were printed by Nestlé. The "only condition", as Victoria put it, was that Nestlé would keep the copyright and, in exchange, they would provide the DEPE with the printed materials. Unlike the DEPE and the SEV itself, Nestlé had unlimited economic and material resources that were channeled through its CSV strategy to fulfil the role of the absent Mexican state. In exchange, Nestlé obtained tangible benefits through the promotion of healthy lifestyles in Veracruz.

In their framing of CSV as the solution to myriad social issues, Porter and Kramer (2011), who have worked closely with Nestlé to validate the efficacy of CSV, depict corporations as charitable entities that can use their "skills, resources, and management capability to lead social progress in ways that even the best-intentioned governmental and social sector organizations can rarely match" (p. 77). In Mexico, Nestlé provides jobs in its factories, development & research centers and headquarters, and undeniably contributes to the economy. However, the extent to which Nestlé's activities in local communities actually benefit the local populations is a subject of debate. For example, a large body of literature has demonstrated how local producers are disadvantaged by Nestlé's control of the coffee market, and how CSV has served more its own interests than those of community development (Charveriat, 2001; Renard, 2010; Renard & Loconto, 2013; Renard & Pérez-Grovas, 2007).

Rose's (2001, p. 6) assertion, that under neoliberalism "society's needs for health" are no longer expected to be solved by the state itself, has been shown to be true in Mexico. The explosion, in the last decade, of programs by corporations that promote healthy lifestyles is a clear example. In this context, Rose claims, the state becomes an "animator". However, what the Mexican case can tell us is that although the state has been reduced, corporate programs could not successfully operate without a *collaborative* state. The work of the SUMA-Nutrir staff, state employees within the SEV, gives us an example of how a specific branch of the state worked, perhaps unwittingly, to expand a corporate bio-political regime. Also, through the words of the SUMA-Nutrir collaborators at the SEV, we can notice that the lack of funding has made state workers more reliant on corporate funding to develop activities and implement policy that would be hard to achieve without public funds.

In December 2018, Nestlé and the newly elected López Obrador administration announced the construction of a new coffee factory in Veracruz. The plant is now open and operating. It is expected that this factory will lead to Mexico outstripping Brazil as the largest producer of Nestlé coffee (Monroy, 2018). In this context, it might not be inappropriate to say, with the history of the Rockefeller Foundation's campaigns and oil corporations in mind (see Chapter 2), that through the work done under Nutrir, Nestlé has also positioned its image among the population of Veracruz to achieve its economic goals there. Victoria was conscious of this issue when she declared that Nestlé "had chosen" to implement Nutrir in Veracruz because they had factories in the state. This fact reminds us of the Rockefeller Foundation's preference for implementing their malaria and hookworm campaigns in the oil-rich Veracruz in the 1920s. Victoria and her colleagues took the risk of partnering with Nestlé, seeking to contribute in the making of 'healthy' Mexicans, perhaps unaware of the fact that, through their committed work, they were aiding the corporate bio-political project. What I want to suggest with the evidence that I have presented here is that the DEPE staff were launched into corporate hands by the absence of the Mexican state.

This chapter offered a from-the-ground view of the complex workings of public–corporate partnerships that aim to make 'healthy' citizens. Together with policies like the *Lineamientos*, the health-promotion programs implemented through these partnerships constitute the discourse of healthy eating deployed to govern food practices in schools. In Chapter 5, I will explore how this discourse is adapted, adopted and resisted in the concrete practices of cooking and sharing food in schools.

Notes

1 SUMA is the acronym for the long name "Somos una comunidad comprometida con una alimentación sana, un manejo adecuado de los residuos, agua para nuestro futuro y la activación física" [We are a community committed with the promotion of healthy eating, responsible water consumption, physical activity and recycling].

2 Victoria was a very articulate woman in her mid-forties who spoke with a profound passion for her work. By the time of my fieldwork in 2016, Victoria had been working in education in Veracruz for nearly 20 years, 10 of which were within the DEPE. She knew the needs, issues, weaknesses, strengths and sociodemographic conditions of each school district in the state. Previously, she had worked as a generalist teacher and as an education adviser within a school district. She was well versed in SEV and teachers' union politics.

3 The program has changed names since then. Today it is called United for Healthy Kids. I will use Nestlé's own abbreviation, U4HK, for this strategy.

4 The Creating Shared Value annual reports of Nestlé detail what CSV does for Nestlé and for the community in Nestlé's key areas. Examples of these reports are listed in the

references as Nestlé (2015) and Nestlé (2019). For a definition of CSV and a brief discussion of the concept, see note 10 below.

5 My discussion of how Corporate Social Responsibility and Creating Shared Value—which I treat as the same thing—work for the benefit of its makers is largely influenced by the views of critical scholars in the field of business ethics (Alcadipani & de Oliveira Medeiros, 2020; Ozkazanc-Pan, 2019; Pearson et al., 2019; Vallentin & Murillo, 2012).

6 I am aware of the risk of depicting Nestlé as a homogenised entity. However, while I do this mainly for purposes of clarity, I also want to highlight the mechanism through which this corporation has advanced its agenda in the name of promoting healthy lifestyles. In making this claim, I want to join the critical conversations about the roles of transnational corporations of different kinds in shaping policy to pursue their interests. I found Benson's and Kirsch's (2010) arguments, and the comments they received on their paper published in the journal *Current Anthropology*, quite provocative. See also Foster (2010).

7 FIA stands for "Ficha Individual Acumulativa", an electronic tool used to collect students' height, weight, medical conditions, socio-economic status and other details.

8 Boiled corn kernels served with mayonnaise, cheese, lime and chilli.

9 For examples from different countries, see Burrows (2012; New Zealand); Friedman (2015; United States and Australia); Mitchinson (2016; Canada); Saldaña-Tejeda (2018; Mexico).

10 Porter and Kramer (2011, p. 66) define creating shared value (CSV) as "policies and operating practices that enhance the competitiveness of a company while simultaneously advancing the economic and social conditions in the communities in which it operates". The difference between corporate social responsibility (CSR) and CSV is, as Porter and Kramer (2011, p. 76) claim, that the former "mostly focus[es] on reputation and have only a limited connection to the business" whereas the latter integrates "company's profitability and competitive position [to] leverage the unique resources and expertise of the company to create economic value". Thus, Claudia said, in adopting a CSV approach to "doing business", Nestlé wanted to take "one step beyond corporate social responsibility that in Mexico is focused on donations, perhaps philanthropy". Nestlé went beyond CSR and implemented "actions that are aligned with our value chain and with Nestlé's strategic areas" to maximize benefit for both society and Nestlé. And "at the heart of Nestlé", Claudia asserted, was nutrition. Aware of the differences between CSR, CSV and philanthropy, I utilise these terms interchangeably here, merely for the purpose of simplicity.

11 The original text in Spanish says: "!Resiste! Evita la tentación y come hasta llegar a casa". An electronic copy of this draft poster was given to me by Mario on the day I interviewed him.

12 The program has changed names in the last five years. Claudia referred to this global strategy that brings together all Nestlé's programs promoting healthy lifestyles among children as Unidos por Niños Saludables [United for Healthy Kids]. I will use Nestlé's own abbreviation, U4HK, for this strategy.

13 The State of Mexico is one of 32 states in Mexico, which I will capitalize to avoid confusion with similar words.

14 Drawing on bio-politics, some scholars have paid attention to the role of numbers in the construction of forms of government. Appadurai (1993, as discussed in Gupta, 2012) sees numbers as government devices deployed to control and organize the social body. Gupta (2012, pp. 158–159), expanding Appadurai's ideas, argues that "enumeration is not merely a tool of political domination" nor a "neutral technology of government". These ideas are relevant here. Similarly, this discussion has benefited from Cházaro's (2008, 2012) studies on the place that tools, measures and demographic statistics had in the political construction of Mexico and the Mexican population in the late nineteenth century.

15 After it was finished in 2013, this factory became Nestlé's largest coffee production facility in the world.
16 DIF stands for "Sistema Nacional de Desarrollo Integral para la Familia" [National System for the Integral Development of Families]. Its aim is to provide welfare for families.

References

Aguilar-Rodríguez, S. (2009). La mesa está servida: Comida y vida cotidiana en el México de mediados del siglo XX [The table is served: Food and daily life in mid-twentieth century Mexico]. *HIB: Revista de Historia Iberoamericana*, 2(2), 52–85. https://dialnet.unirioja.es/servlet/articulo?codigo=3620992.

Alcadipani, R., & de Oliveira Medeiros, C. R. (2020). When corporations cause harm: A critical view of corporate social irresponsibility and corporate crimes. *Journal of Business Ethics*, 167(2), 285–297. https://doi.org/10.1007/s10551-019-04157-0.

Appadurai, A. (2001). Deep democracy: Urban governmentality and the horizon of politics. *Environment and Urbanization*, 13(2), 23–43. https://doi.org/10.1177/095624780101300203.

Arvizú Martínez, O., Polo Oteyza, E., & Shamah Levy, T. (eds.). (2015). *Qué y cómo comemos los Mexicanos. Consumo de alimentos en la población urbana* [*What and how Mexicans eat. Food consumption in the urban population*]. INSP/FUNSALUD/Fondo Nestlé para la Nutrición.

Benson, P., & Kirsch, S. (2010). Capitalism and the politics of resignation. *Current Anthropology*, 51(4), 459–486. https://doi.org/10.1086/653091.

Burrows, L. (2012). Pedagogizing families through obesity discourse. In J. Wright & V. Harwood (eds.), *Biopolitics and the 'obesity epidemic': Governing bodies* (pp. 135–148). Routledge.

Charveriat, C. (2001). *Bitter coffee: How the poor are paying for the slump in coffee prices.* Oxfam GB, http://hdl.handle.net/10546/114002.

Cházaro, L. (2008). Regímenes e instrumentos de medición: Las medidas de los cuerpos y del territorio nacional en el siglo XIX en México [Regimens and instruments of measurement: Measuring bodies and national territory in 19th century Mexico]. *Nuevo Mundo, Mundos Nuevos*, 8(2008). https://doi.org/10.4000/nuevomundo.14052.

Cházaro, L. (2012). Las estadísticas médicas y la investigación científica [Medical statistics and scientific research]. *Ciencia. Revista de la Academia Mexicana de Ciencias*, 63 (April – June), 56–63.

Crane, A., Palazzo, G., Spence, L. J., & Matten, D. (2014). Contesting the value of "Creating Shared Value". *California Management Review*, 56(2), 130–153. https://doi.org/10.1525/cmr.2014.56.2.130.

Drewnowski, A., Caballero, B., Das, J. K., French, J., Prentice, A. M., Fries, L. R., van Koperen, T. M., Klassen-Wigger, P., & Rolls, B. J. (2018). Novel public–private partnerships to address the double burden of malnutrition. *Nutrition Reviews* 76(11), 805–821. https://doi.org/10.1093/nutrit/nuy035.

Escobar, A. (2011). *Encountering development: The making and unmaking of the third world* (2nd ed.). Princeton University Press.

Foster, R. J. (2010). Corporate oxymorons and the anthropology of corporations. *Dialectical Anthropology*, 34(1), 95–102. https://doi.org/10.1007/s10624-009-9126-5.

Foucault, M. (2007). *Security, territory, population. Lectures at the Collège de France 1977–1978*, translated by G. Burchell, Picador.

Foucault, M. (2008). *The birth of biopolitics: Lectures at the Collège De France 1978–1979* translated by G. Burchell, Picador.

Friedman, M. (2015). Mother blame, fat shame, and moral panic: "Obesity" and child welfare. *Fat Studies*, 4(1), 14–27. https://doi.org/10.1080/21604851.2014.927209.

Gupta, A. (2012). *Red tape: Bureaucracy, structural violence and poverty in India*. Duke University Press.

Herrick, C. (2009). Shifting blame/selling health: Corporate social responsibility in the age of obesity. *Sociology of Health & Illness*, 31(1), 51–65. https://doi.org/10.1111/j.1467-9566.2008.01121.x.

Leone, L., Ling, T., Baldassarre, L., Barnett, L. M., Capranica, L., & Pesce, C. (2015). Corporate responsibility for childhood physical activity promotion in the UK. *Health Promotion International*, 1–14. https://doi.org/10.1093/heapro/dav051.

Lineamientos 2010 (Acuerdo mediante el cual se establecen los lineamientos generales para el expendio o distribución de alimentos y bebidas en los establecimientos de consumo escolar de los planteles de educación básica [General guidelines for the distribution or sales of food and drinks by retailers within basic education schools]) (2010). Diario Oficial de la Federación: Órgano del Gobierno Constitucional de los Estados Unidos Mexicanos.

Lineamientos 2014 (Acuerdo mediante el cual se establecen los lineamientos generales para el expendio y distribución de alimentos y bebidas preparados y procesados en las escuelas del Sistema Educativo Nacional [Guidelines for the sales and distribution of prepared and processed food and drinks in the Mexican national education system]) (2014). Diario Oficial de la Federación: Órgano del Gobierno Constitucional de los Estados Unidos Mexicanos.

Mitchinson, W. (2016). Mother blaming and obesity: An alternative perspective. In J. Ellison, D. McPhail, & W. Mitchinson (eds.), *Obesity in Canda: Critical perspectives* (pp. 187–217). University of Toronto Press.

Monroy, J. (2018). Nestlé invertirá 154 mdd para nueva planta en Veracruz [Nestlé will invest 154 mdd to build a new factory in Veracruz]. *El Economista*. https://www.eleconomista.com.mx/empresas/Nestle-invertira-154-mdd-para-nueva-planta-en-Veracruz-20181218-0166.html.

Nestlé (2015). *Nestlé in society: Creating Shared Value and meeting our commitments 2014. Full report*. http://www.nestle.com/asset-library/documents/library/documents/corporate_social_responsibility/nestle-csv-full-report-2014-en.pdf.

Nestlé (2019). *Creating Shared Value and meeting our commitments 2018. Progress report*. https://www.nestle.com/sites/default/files/asset-library/documents/library/documents/corporate_social_responsibility/creating-shared-value-report-2018-en.pdf.

Nestlé México (2013). *Recetario regional: Comiendo bien a lo Veracruz-sano [Regional cookbook: Eating well in a healthy-Veracruz-style]*. Nestlé México.

Nestlé México (2015). 675,00 niños veracruzanos han sido capacitados en hábitos saludables por NUTRIR de NESTLÉ [675.00 children from Veracruz have been trained in healthy habits by NUTRIR from NESTLÉ]. Retrieved 13 October 2015 from https://www.nestle.com.mx/media/pressreleases/675000-nios-veracruzanos-han-sido-capacitados-en-hbitos-saludables-por-nutrir-de-nestl.

Nestlé México (2016). *Recetario regional volumen 2: Comiendo bien a lo Veracruz-sano [Regional cookbook volume 2: Eating well in a healthy-Veracruz-style]* (2nd ed.). Nestlé México.

Ozkazanc-Pan, B. (2019). CSR as gendered neocoloniality in the Global South. *Journal of Business Ethics*, 160(4), 851–864. https://doi.org/10.1007/s10551-018-3798-1.

Pearson, Z., Ellingrod, S., Billo, E., & McSweeney, K. (2019). Corporate social responsibility and the reproduction of (neo)colonialism in the Ecuadorian Amazon. *The*

100 *Corporatizing Healthy Eating*

Extractive Industries and Society, 6(3), 881–888. https://doi.org/10.1016/j.exis.2019.05.016.

Porter, M. E., & Kramer, M. R. (2011). Creating Shared Value. *Harvard Business Review*, 89(1–2), 62–77.

Renard, M.-C. (2010). In the name of conservation: CAFE practices and fair trade in Mexico. *Journal of Business Ethics*, 92(2), 287–299. https://doi.org/10.1007/s10551-010-0584-0.

Renard, M.-C., & Loconto, A. (2013). Competing logics in the further standardization of fair trade: SEAL and the símbolo de pequeños productores. *The International Journal of Sociology of Agriculture and Food*, 20(1), 51–68. https://doi.org/10.48416/ijsaf.v20i1.201.

Renard, M.-C., & Pérez-Grovas, V. (2007). Fair trade coffee in Mexico: At the center of the debates. In L. T. Raynolds, D. L. Murray, & J. Wilkinson (eds.), *Fair trade: The challenges of transforming globalization* (pp. 138–156). Routledge.

Rose, N. (2001). The politics of life itself. *Theory, Culture & Society*, 18(6), 1–30. https://doi.org/10.1177/02632760122052020.

Ruckert, A., & Labonté, R. (2014). Public–private partnerships (PPPs) in global health: The good, the bad and the ugly. *Third World Quarterly*, 35(9), 1598–1614. https://doi.org/10.1080/01436597.2014.970870.

Saldaña-Tejeda, A. (2018). Mitochondrial mothers of a fat nation: Race, gender and epigenetics in obesity research on Mexican mestizos. *BioSocieties*, 13(2), 434–452. https://doi.org/10.1057/s41292-017-0078-8.

Semple, K. (2017, April 16). Javier Duarte, Mexican ex-Governor accused of diverting money, is captured. *The New York Times*. https://www.nytimes.com/2017/04/16/world/americas/mexico-javier-duarte-captured.html.

Shamir, R. (2004). The de-radicalization of corporate social responsibility. *Critical Sociology*, 30(3), 669–689. https://doi.org/10.1163/1569163042119831.

Sharma, A. (2008). *Logics of empowerment: Development, gender, and governance in neoliberal India*. University of Minnesota Press.

Vallentin, S., & Murillo, D. (2012). Governmentality and the politics of CSR. *Organization*, 19(6), 825–843. https://doi.org/10.1177/1350508411426183.

Vander Schee, C. J., & Boyles, D. (2010). 'Exergaming,' corporate interests and the crisis discourse of childhood obesity. *Sport, Education and Society*, 15(2), 169–185. https://doi.org/10.1080/13573321003683828.

Watson, K. (2016). Disappearing Duarte: Where is Veracruz's governor? *BBC Mexico*. http://www.bbc.com/news/world-latin-america-37776955.

5 Beyond Policy
Everyday Cooking in Schools

Victoria, the leader of the healthy eating program SUMA-Nutrir (see Chapter 4), was a student at Emiliano Zapata Primary School in the 1980s. Having had grown in Santa Rosa, she knew the community and the school well. For this reason, Victoria selected Emiliano Zapata Primary School as a "pilot school" to test various programs before implementing them across the state. SUMA-Nutrir was one of them. Her connections—some of the teachers in the school had been her teachers, and they were friends now—and local knowledge provided Victoria certainty about commitment in the implementation. This also afforded her direct communication about the program's progress.

Benito Juárez Primary School was chosen as a "pilot school" for SUMA-Nutrir because of its size. The school had a catchment of nearly 1,000 students—outstanding for a public primary school in the state of Veracruz. Corporate-sponsored programs of different kinds had already taken place, or were ongoing during my fieldwork, in the school. Its political relevance also made Benito Juárez Primary School an organization to be approached for the implementation of programs (Chapter 2). The school leadership considered they were one of the best primary schools in Veracruz. As the principal, Susana, used to proudly claim, they were "even better than private schools". Benito Juárez Primary School was certainly well resourced in terms of infrastructure, economic resources and staff.

SUMA-Nutrir was rolled out in both schools in the 2011–2012 school year (August–July). During this year, Emiliano Zapata and Benito Juárez primary schools reported to the Dirección de Educación Primaria Estatal (DEPE) and were occasionally visited by Victoria and her team. At the end of the school year, in July 2012, the DEPE organized in partnership with Nestlé a series of events around the state where the "pilot schools" presented how they were promoting healthy lifestyles. These events, called "Jornadas de Cierre", aimed to collect feedback to improve the program, hear from the experiences of teachers, parents and students and prove that SUMA-Nutrir had had an impact. One of the main outcomes of these events was the first volume of the *Comiendo Bien a lo Veracruzsano* cookbook (Chapter 4).[1]

A year before, the *Lineamientos 2010*, a school food policy, had been launched. The DEPE oversaw its implementation, through the school districts, across the primary schools in Veracruz. Both Benito Juárez and Emiliano Zapata primary

DOI: 10.4324/9781003356264-5

schools, as I discussed in Chapter 1, tried to enact the nutritional recommendations of this policy. Together, the *Lineamientos* and SUMA-Nutrir constituted a powerful tool for regulating food in schools. The constant supervision and support provided to "pilot schools" yielded some results. It was hard, but schools managed to, momentarily, change some of their foods on offer. In 2013 and 2014, Emiliano Zapata and Benito Juárez primary schools were characterized as "successful" examples of how healthy lifestyles initiatives can generate positive change in food practices. Victoria was particularly enthusiastic of this idea. This is why she suggested I take these two schools as sites of observation during my fieldwork in 2016.

The everyday working of healthy lifestyles in schools has been largely overlooked. The focus on "impact" and "effectiveness" has reduced schools and the people within them to numbers; numbers that are used to *prove* that healthy lifestyles initiatives work. In this chapter, I present a series of ethnographic encounters that shed light on the unreliable meanings and significant tensions of 'healthy lifestyles' in the economically rough, and highly politicized, contexts of Benito Juárez and Emiliano Zapata primary schools. From this vantage point, I expose issues that, deliberatively or not, have been unheeded by the voices who claim that schools are "ideal" spaces to 'fight' obesity. The actors who have had the right to speak about obesity have proposed solutions in line with global scientific evidence. However, sometimes they have been unable, or reluctant, to see that that evidence might not match the needs of the Mexican society. The solutions therefore are significantly de-contextualized.

'Healthy lifestyles', as this book has shown so far, has generated an array of practices that, underpinned by the energy balance and shared responsibility discourses, have reduced food to an object that must be quantified in the name of health. The *Lineamientos* and SUMA-Nutrir have played a significant role in this process. Beyond the reductionist association of food and health promoted by the *dispositif of healthy lifestyles* however, the place and function of food within Mexican society are rather complex. Food, or the 'informal' sale of food to be more precise, also has a central role in the Mexican economy.[2] Food, *real food*,[3] is cooked, many times from scratch from a variety of ingredients, by women under, many times, difficult conditions. Food in schools, as this chapter demonstrates, also serves different, often competing purposes.[4] Notably, real food, and all its associated practices, functions as a subsistence mechanism and an expression of care.

This chapter situates schools as historical and political spaces (see Chapters 1 and 2). The aim is to show how internal and local politics, funding—or the lack thereof, staffing and culture shape the practices of food in these spaces.[5] The remainder of this chapter is divided in three sections. The first section is focused on Benito Juárez Primary School and the second one on Emiliano Zapata Primary School. In these sections, I first contextualize the schools to then discuss how food was prepared and sold in each of them. I decided to have a separate discussion for each school to emphasize difference. My aim, however, is far from arguing for one 'ideal' form of school food management. Instead, I seek to expose how macro- and micro-economic and political issues and culture shape the practices of cooking, selling and eating in each school. Food cannot be reduced to 'energy'. If school food regulations are to be more effective, they need to expand their narrow view on food and its association with health. More attention needs to be given to the cultured and economical process of cooking and to the people (women) who arduously make food exist. The last section of this chapter is devoted to discussing these ideas.

Benito Juárez Primary School

Benito Juárez Primary School opened its doors in the 2008–2009 school year. The school started with 40 students and two staff members: Susana, the principal, and Diana, the vice-principal. Two groups, each of 20 students, were taught by them. Both the student enrolment and the number of staff increased considerably thereafter. The school had been built by the developers of Paso de Leones. Similar to what occurred in other "developments" constructed between 2000 and 2010, during the so-called housing boom, the school infrastructure was left unfinished.[6] To equip the school, Susana had to raise funds from parents, businesses, education authorities and, especially, political parties. In only two years, the school became well-resourced. Susana's connections and the politically strategic location of the school, as I mentioned at the beginning of Chapter 2, had much to do with this.

Susana was in her early 30s in 2016; very young to be a principal.[7] She started her career in the education system in Veracruz in 2003, immediately after graduating, as a principal. This is not common. She was truly "well-connected" and strategically positioned. This, to an extent, benefited the school and the community. Benito Juárez Primary School was situated in a large square bordered by a

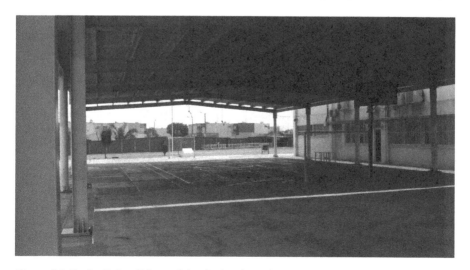

Figure 5.1 Benito Juárez Primary School: view from the amphitheater. Photo by the author.

redbrick wall. Inside the walls, there was one large four-story building containing 18 classrooms, offices and the school library. All the rooms in this building were air-conditioned. Behind this building there was a large covered main court and an amphitheater. Nutrilandia, the space where food was produced and sold, was located next to the amphitheater (see Figure 2.1). 12 surveillance cameras were strategically situated around the school. All these features were uncommon in public primary schools in Veracruz.

Benito Juárez Primary School was a "double-shift school"[8] working from 8 am to 6 pm; it had a morning (8 am to 12:30 pm) and an afternoon shift (2 pm to 6 pm). For these two shifts there were 59 school staff members, including the principal, vice-principal, six curriculum advisers, two secretaries, four physical education teachers, two librarians, two English teacher, six cleaners and 35 generalist teachers. The two cleaners and the English teachers were paid from the profits of food sales profits and from the "voluntary" parents' fees. In the "morning shift" there were 18 groups of students (three groups of each grade) and in the "afternoon shift" there were 15. According to staff, most students were lower-class, while some came from poor families and a few were slightly better-off.

Public–corporate partnerships were common in the school. Noteworthy was the partnership established between the school and TenarisTamsa, a global manufacturer of steel pipelines based in Veracruz. This partnership started in 2010. As part of it, Susana and Diana participated in a diploma called LISTO, launched by TenarisTamsa to "empower" school leaders in Veracruz to drive change.[9] In 2012, Benito Juárez Primary School joined the program Escuelas de Excelencia [Schools of Excellence], also sponsored by TenarisTamsa and other corporations. This program involved the entire school. Its aim was to "teach" teachers how "teach better". Like most of the corporate-sponsored programs launched in the last decade, Escuelas de Excelencia provided no material or economic resources to the school. It was all about "empowering" through discourse. To become a 'school of excellence', staff at Benito Juárez Primary School had to endure the constant surveillance of an external "expert", a "coach", in Susana's words, trained in education management in Mexico City and overseas.

Gina, the coach, oversaw the school's functioning for a year. Teachers had to shape their planning and teaching to Gina's recommendations. Classrooms were rearranged to foster "efficient learning". "It was a horrible external assessment!", Susana told me. Pedagogies in the classroom started to be modelled by industrial relations based on productivity. "All the lesson plans had to be verified by Gina and if she was not happy with them, teachers had to do them again. After six months, teachers hated her!". Teachers did not see much benefit in the program. It was more work. But Susana, who was convinced of its advantages, pushed it through. She wanted to demonstrate that "public schools could be as good as their private counterparts". To prove this, the school needed to perform well in the national standardized test. The physical infrastructure was an issue Benito Juárez Primary School had sorted. Yet it needed to be more efficient in teaching and learning to achieve these goals. Corporate programs offered 'help' with this. The deep penetration of corporate rationales and the eagerness to be represented as a 'model' public school also framed the practices of cooking and selling food in Nutrilandia.

The name Nutrilandia had been added to the cooperativa escolar [school cooperative] as part of the implementation of SUMA-Nutrir. "Nutrilandia" results from the combination of the Spanish word *nutrición* [nutrition] and the suffix *-landia*, which makes reference to land in English. Nutrilandia refers to the "land of nutrition", an idea framed under a narrow view of food and health that was difficult to achieve in the day-to-day. Feeding nearly 1,000 students with affordable, tasty and nutritious foods was not an easy task. At the time of my fieldwork, Elena, Nutrilandia's operator, was in charge of preparing and selling food in the school under an "outsourcing model", as teachers called it. This form of food management was fairly recent in the school. From 2008 to 2012, the food management was anchored to the *Reglamento 1982* (see Chapter 2). In those four years, a group of mothers delivered homemade foods to the school and teachers and the kids sold them together as an educational exercise. The aim, as teachers and the school leadership put it, was to use the cooperativa escolar to "teach students the value of money and how to make transactions". However, as student enrolment and teachers' workload increased, Benito Juárez Primary School had to change this form of managing school food, as is discussed below.

In 2016, the *Lineamientos* had been out for six years, and had been amended once. Yet all the school staff still spoke about food organization in terms of cooperativas escolares. Most of the staff considered that cooperativas should ideally be run by teachers and students. They in fact expressed "concern" for having a third party managing the production and sale of food in the school. No one was aware that the *Lineamientos* 2010 and 2014 had eliminated the cooperativas escolares and granted permission to schools to subcontract third parties, like Elena, to prepare and sell food within the school.

After winning the food-provider bid, Elena became Nutrilandia's administrator in 2014. In a "thorough competition", as Susana described it to me, several women, all of the them school mothers, presented their menus to be judged by the school community. Elena said that she won the bid because, unlike the other women, she offered "*light* options" ("light" said in English). Elena, aged around 40, was married and had two daughters, one still studying at Benito Juárez Primary School. Elena and her husband both worked at Nutrilandia, and their two daughters sometimes helped them after school. Elena was the manager and head cook, instructing her three female employees on what and how to cook. Her husband stocked ingredients, received the deliveries and delivered food to teachers. Nutrilandia was a small family business.

Benito Juárez Primary School's authorities decided to put food sales in the hands of an external contractor to minimize the "wasted" time devoted by teachers to selling food. The LISTO and Escuelas de Excelencia programs were demanding and sought to maximize efficiency. Putting the provisioning of food into external hands also decreased financial risk for the school. Food sales could generate good income one week but be bad the next week, especially if ultra-processed products were not for sale. Outsourcing the production and sale of food, however, transferred the risk to a third party, which would pay a daily fee to the school in exchange for being permitted to do business. This was more convenient and profitable for the school. This profit-driven model of food provisioning, however, had some negative consequences for children.

Profits from food sales had to pay for both Elena and the school. Potato chips and cookies represented convenience and a good profit margin for Elena. These products also brought other benefits for Nutrilandia. In exchange for selling their ultra-processed products, corporations provide cooperativas escolares with tables, fridges, chairs and other tools that are hard for Mexican schools to afford otherwise. *Masa*-based foods, like *empanadas* and *quesadillas*, were also widely sold in Benito Juárez Primary School. However, their labor-intensive nature made them less profitable than readily available ultra-processed products. *Quesadillas* were the most expensive of the four options (potato chips, cookies, *quesadillas* and *empanadas*) more widely offered in the schools. The cost of cookies and potato chips was 10 pesos per packet. The price of each *empanada* was 6 pesos, but to get a *quesadilla* students needed to pay 12 pesos, which partly inhibited their purchase. Children also said two *empanadas* were "more filling" than one *quesadilla*.

Elena paid the school 1 peso per child per day as part of her contract. Overall, the school earned around 900 pesos per day, an amount of money that schools like Emiliano Zapata Primary School had only dreamed of. However, this money, which translated into a benefit for the school, came at the price of allowing kids to buy as many ultra-processed products as they could afford. While I am not judging whether this action is good or bad, I do want to raise the point that, in this case, policy compliance became a simulation. Elena, for example, always tried to make it clear that Nutrilandia's food was "healthy". However, her speech about her commitment to "favoring fruit consumption" and "halting fats" contrasted with the standing rack full of Sabritas—PepsiCo's chips brand in Mexico—and packages of sweet baked goods from BIMBO. These products were sold during the break even though the *Lineamientos* banned them from schools.

The school leadership knew these products were being sold even when they should not. However, they allowed it because of the profit it raised for the school. This is the kind of issue that makes the practices around food in Mexican schools an interesting expression of gastro-politics (Appadurai, 1981). But I do not want to be misunderstood. There is not anything bad with Elena and the school profiting from school food. Actually, that profit was very useful for both parties. Food income, together with the parents' fees, paid for the salaries of the English teachers and two cleaners, and supplied the funds that helped the school with a myriad services and maintenance requirements. In addition, Nutrilandia's revenue financed the livelihood of Elena's family.

So, Nutrilandia's profit-driven food sales model produced revenue for the school and for Elena, yet these profits came at a cost. Teachers were aware that a business model like Nutrilandia's required sacrificing the quality of food for convenient, profitable products. Teachers were critical of this issue. Carla, a middle-class, single woman in her late 20s, was very critical of the food options at Nutrilandia. During our interview, she constantly emphasized her dislike for what was sold at the school, and for *masa*-based foods in general. Noticing her insistence in negatively judging Nutrilandia's food and management, I pushed Carla on whether she considered that the products sold were "good options". Laughing loudly, she said:

> Elena (laughs), Elena is not going to listen to this conversation, right? (Brief silence) Definitely, no! I mean, they try to have a balanced menu... But as I've said, there's not enough time. [Products] need to be convenient... they *need to be sold easily* [her emphasis], because many times healthy food [*lo sano*] is not sold as quickly as other products. Elena's clients are kids, and children want sweet things, fried things [*fritangas*], processed snacks [*chucherías*]... So, if they only had a menu with healthy options [*cosas saludables*], they would need to educate their clients, and that would take a long time...

As can be seen, Carla did not agree with the food options at Nutrilandia. Nonetheless, she justified their availability due to their convenience and profitability, which related to the school's managerial model. At the same time, she offered a moral judgement of the students, assigning them to the category of nutritionally "uneducated". Susana had a similar perspective. She also made students responsible for the "unhealthy" food options offered in the school. "[Healthy] products are not sold. Kids don't eat them", Susana emphasized, describing the multiple efforts made by the school to encourage 'healthy' eating in the school. She continued:

> we started offering scrambled eggs with ham... guess what? They didn't eat them. Kids didn't eat the eggs and didn't eat the servings of chopped apple either... The kids don't have the culture [of eating 'healthy']. So, since the cooperativa is a business, the managers end up selling what the client asks for. And what does the client ask for? Well, you've already seen it: *picadas, empanadas, gordas, quesadillas*, that is what the children ask for. So, what we do is that when I realize, when I see that the cooperativa is selling lots of chips, I tell them: "Be careful, *eh*! You're selling lots of chips, what's going on? Don't sell too many chips. Replace them".

Like Carla, Susana also categorically deemed both ultra-processed products and *masa*-based foods as equally "unhealthy". In this conception, handmade *empanadas, quesadillas* and *picadas* are 'unhealthy' because *masa* is the main ingredient and because they contain, to a more or less extent, some form of fat.[10] For both Carla and Susana, the food offered within the school—regardless of whether it had been handmade onsite from known ingredients, or simply stocked by PepsiCo and BIMBO salespersons—was overall "unhealthy". An ideal school meal, from their perspective, should be composed of salads, fruit or sandwiches. The school had indeed offered some of these options between 2008 and 2010 in a set menu, which included an apple, a white-bread ham-and-yellow-cheese sandwich and a bottled juice. Yet, as many teachers told me, this initiative did not work, mostly because of the students' fondness for *masa* and because of the "lack of commitment" by their parents towards healthy eating.

In line with the opinion of many of my interviewees across different sites, Carla and Susana included *masa*-based foods in the "junk food" category, together with industrial potato chips, cookies and candies. This is an example of how the *dispositif of healthy lifestyles* has worked to stigmatize foods that have been part of the Mexican diet for decades or even centuries. While the nutritional messages spread through policies and programs have not explicitly categorized all *masa*-based foods as 'unhealthy', they have proposed to limit, reduce or avoid their consumption.

Another point shared between Carla and Susana is their conception of students as clients. Nutrilandia offered multiple food options that students could choose from. The students who rushed eagerly to Nutrilandia as the break bell rang could exchange their money for a variety of ultra-processed products and handmade foods. However, as happens when profit is the ultimate aim of a business, not every student in the school became a client during the break. Students who neither brought food from home nor had money for food at Nutrilandia were left with an empty stomach. Many times, other students fed these children, sharing the food they had bought in the school or brought from home. The school break time was time for consumption, but also for sharing.

Feeding children in schools is doubtless complicated. Taste, labor, nutritional standards and national and local economic conditions are in constant tension. Research on food practices in schools around the world has contributed to the understanding of these connections. For example, Poppendieck (2010, pp. 44–60) shows that the elimination of the school-food subsidy in the United States in the 1980s demanded that school food "operate like a business". With increasing pressure on food revenue, school administrators introduced "branded items" and ultra-processed products "purchased in bulk" and replaced "employees with cooking skills" for "less-skilled workers" who only had to unpack, heat and serve frozen foods. Cost reductions translated into higher revenue. To justify the introduction of ultra-processed products, Poppendieck claims, school administrators adopted the discourse that highlighted the 'nutritional' qualities of those foods (see also Levine, 2008).

Is school food in Mexico being pushed in the same direction? If I have learned anything from history, I would say, yes. However, from the same history I would also claim that there are multiple cultural conditions that would give the corporatization of school food in Mexico a particular flavor. The presence of handmade foods in a deeply "corporatized" school like Benito Juárez Primary School perhaps proves this point. Depicting the practices around food in Nutrilandia as merely profit-driven would contradict the theoretical tenets underpinning this research. While Nutrilandia always sought to maximize revenue, Elena and her workers also put great effort into handmaking tasty foods. Ultra-processed products were easy, convenient products that did not require labor to be transformed into revenue. In contrast, making *empanadas* and *quesadillas*, which were consumed in large quantities by the children and some teachers, required cooking skills and hours of intense labor.

Benito Juárez Primary School embodied what I call a "corporatized" school.[11] Beyond the moral judgements of the school staff, whom I have no doubt acted with the best intentions in difficult circumstances, this interpretation arose from the enterprise-logic manifest in the school's management. While it would be mistaken to state that all staff at Benito Juárez Primary School aided this project, it could be suggested that Susana, perhaps unwittingly, directed the establishment of corporate-like management in the school. Her desire to make Benito Juárez Primary School an archetype of a "good public school", combined with the skills that she acquired through multiple corporate-funded programs, pushed Susana to implement a series of accountability mechanisms and an enterprise management in the school. This is reflected in her idea of the cooperativa escolar as a business and the students as clients, which also influenced the practices of cooking and selling food in the school.

Emiliano Zapata Primary School

Emiliano Zapata Primary School is strategically located in the middle of Santa Rosa, between a kindergarten and a communal space called La Casa del Campesino [The Peasant's House]. This space is owned by the local peasant coalition and contain a large room and a covered patio. The school is bounded by an old fence. It comprises six classrooms, one multi-media classroom, one kitchen and the principal's office. When it was built in the 1960s, the school comprised only three classrooms and a large yard. These rooms have high-ceilings and big windows on both sides to enable breezes to flow through. The walls and the tiles show their age. In 2016, these rooms were used as the kitchen, the multi-media room and a

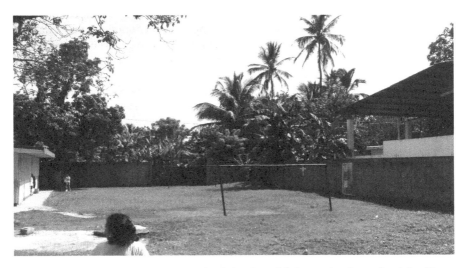

Figure 5.2 Emiliano Zapata Primary School. La Casa del Campesino is on the right. Photo by the author.

classroom. The classrooms built later are smaller. In 2016, there were seven student groups: two first-grade groups and one group for each of the other grades (second to sixth grade). Since there were seven groups but only six classrooms available, the school used the building at La Casa del Campesino as an extra classroom.

Santa Rosa is not the official name of the community where the school is located. The official name of this place is Carmen Serdán. The town was named Carmen Serdán in 1932, after a prominent member of the Veracruz League of Agrarian Communities, a group of radical insurgents who pursued land reform in this region during the 1920s and 1930s.[12] The name change reflected the transition in administrative status from a private holding, a hacienda, to a community where peasants benefited from the agrarian reform carried out by Lázaro Cárdenas (see Chapter 2). Yet in 2016 people continued to call the place by its previous hacienda name: Santa Rosa. The name Carmen Serdán was used for very specific, mostly official, purposes.

Neither time nor reforms have altered the dependency of Santa Rosa, and other nearby towns, on the sugar cane industry. The lives, and the cooking and eating practices, of the school community revolved around the sugar cane cycle. During "high season" (harvest time between November and May) they earned around 100 pesos per day, either as canecutters or as truck drivers. During the "low season" (June–October), families struggled to make ends meet. While sugar cane grew, fathers usually worked as day laborers in nearby plantations or caught *mojarras* [a white fish] from the river and sold them along the roads. Mothers were mostly housewives but also contributed to sustaining their households by selling food, cleaning or sewing. NAFTA, as I have described in Chapters 1 and 2, has exacerbated unemployment and migration in the region.

At the time of my fieldwork, approximately 140 students attended Emiliano Zapata Primary School. They were of varying socio-economic status but predominantly poor. The school staff comprised the principal, seven teachers, one English teacher, two physical education teachers, one arts teacher, one special education teacher, one IT teacher, one cleaner and four cooks. The teachers and the principal had worked there for at least 10 years. Only the teachers, the cleaner, the principal and the four cooks worked five days a week. The other teaching staff came to the school once or twice a week. The cooks were paid 80 pesos per day out of the money collected from the food sales.

The kitchen was set up in 2008, when the school joined the Programa de Escuelas de Tiempo Completo (PETC)—a federal program aimed at "improving" academic achievement in Mexican schools through the extension of the school day. In Veracruz, children attend primary school from 8:00 am to 1:00 pm. The PETC extended the school day until 3:30 pm. The implications of the program in the workings of schools were significant. Teachers were required to work a longer day. Schools also needed to provide students with more food throughout the day, but they lacked the infrastructure and economic and human resources to do so. The federal funds attached to the PETC were distributed to state governments. In Veracruz, however, funding was diverted.[13] Teachers in Emiliano Zapata Primary

School essentially donated their labor to stay in the program. They hoped funds would reach the school at some point.

As part of the PETC schools needed to provide to breakfast at 10:30 am and lunch at 1:00 pm to students. Emiliano Zapata Primary School lacked the infrastructure to do this. In 2008, when the PETC started in the school, a group of women sold food—mostly homemade *masa*-based foods—during the break at 10:30 am. The school community decided to convert one classroom into the kitchen. This, however, created a serious problem: the school lost one classroom. To solve this issue, the school authorities borrowed La Casa del Campesino and adapted it into a classroom. Rosalba, an experienced teacher who acted as principal between 2007 and 2013, was fundamental in establishing the kitchen. She organized parents and sought "alternative" ways to obtain funding. Luckily, in 2008, Rosalba's brother was the local councilor in Santa Rosa. Kinship connections translated into material help for the school. "But don't tell this to others, *eh*!", Rosalba said when she told me about this experience.

In an ideal world, the school would have received funding and SEV planners would have designed the kitchen and dining area. However, knowing that this would never occur, the school community became both the funders and the designers of these spaces. They selected the classroom next to the multi-media room because of its tactical location. Its door faced the main patio, so teachers envisaged making another door at the back to allow students to go directly into the dining area. I witnessed the results of this ingenious design. The kitchen's front and rear doors facilitated a multidirectional flow of students: they came in through the front door; interacted with people while receiving their breakfast; and left for the dining area through the rear door. If their serving had not satisfied their appetite, students could come back in again through the same door.[14]

Feeding children in a school requires more than having a physical space where food can be prepared. Ingredients and people to convert them into foods are also needed. Between 2008 and 2010, the school community established a participatory scheme where four mothers from each grade group helped operate the kitchen on a weekly basis. Under this system, the four mothers had to devote several hours of unpaid labor per day to source ingredients, cook, serve food and clean the kitchen. The price per meal, 6 pesos, only reflected the cost of ingredients. It did not work. From the beginning of the 2010–2011 school year, the breakfast's price increased to 8 pesos, to include 2 pesos to pay the salaries for four women to work permanently in the kitchen. It was then that Doña Martha, Beatriz, Moni and Angela—the *Doñitas*, as I usually referred to them—became cooks for the modest wage of 60 pesos per five hours of intense labor.

In 2016, the school functioned from 8:00 am to 2:00 pm. Funds from the PETC never reached the school. It was impossible for teachers to work for "free" until 3:00 pm and to find the money to feed the students twice. Only one meal was offered at 10:30 am. The fee for breakfast was 10 pesos. The cooks' salary also increased to 80 pesos per shift. Cooking began at 8:00 am and finished around 1:00 pm, after the kitchen and dining area had been thoroughly cleaned. A set of old plastic tables, a makeshift stove, a microwave, a blender, a domestic fridge and heavily used kitchenware were the sparse tools that the cooks used to "make miracles", as they called the action of cooking with limited materials and economic resources.

The four Doñitas were wise women and adroit cooks. Doña Martha, in her 60s, had a long history at Emiliano Zapata Primary School. Hailing from the state of Hidalgo, she and her husband came to Santa Rosa in the late 1970s looking for work in sugar farming.[15] Her three sons attended Emiliano Zapata Primary School in the 1980s. She became the school janitor, paid daily from school funds. From the late 1990s, she sold *masa*-based foods at the school for several years, until the kitchen was set up. Her robust arms embodied hard work and cooking knowledges. Beatriz and Moni were in their late 30s. Each had a child in sixth grade and had been working in the school kitchen for about five years. Their husbands were day-laborers in the cane fields. Angela, the youngest in her late 20s, had two children at school. She had been a cook at Emiliano Zapata Primary School for about two years. Of the four cooks, Doña Martha was the most "affluent" since her sons were already in their 30s and her husband was a permanent blue-collar worker in the sugar mill. The other three women struggled to make ends meet. The 80 pesos they made a day were vital in their households.

Apart from the cooks, the kitchen activities also directly involved Olga, a teacher, and Rafa, the janitor. Olga was responsible for sourcing ingredients and, together with the cooks, devising the menu. Both tasks were done on a daily basis. It could not have been otherwise because the decision depended on the amount of money raised from the breakfast the previous day. Olga bought the ingredients in Zamora, a larger town ten minutes from Santa Rosa. She was always chasing the best prices and usually the menu depended on the cost of vegetables. Rafa helped in the kitchen, collecting the students' 10-peso contribution classroom-by-classroom each morning, going to the local grocery store to buy last-minute ingredients and helping with the cooking if required.

In spite of the launching of the *Lineamientos*, in 2016 food in Emiliano Zapata Primary School continued to be organized under the cooperativa escolar model. The kitchen could not operate without the funds supplied by the sale of drinks and other products. Principal Andrés managed the drinks sales by himself. Every week, he received six cases of bottled water, distributed by a Coca-Cola delivery, sold them to the students from his office and administered the limited revenue (see Chapter 6). The seven teachers were responsible for selling various products at the breaktime. Two teams of teachers sourced, prepared and sold the products for one week each team. Trying to comply with the *Lineamientos*' and SUMA-Nutrir's directions, sliced fruits with lime and chili powder, were usually available on Monday and Tuesday. On the rest of the weekdays, hot cakes, nachos and candies were sold. However, this was not a rule. Most of the times all products were sold simultaneously. Every morning when the break bell rang, the team members prepared what was required. Frozen hot cakes were unpacked, heated up in the microwave and wrapped in a cloth to keep them warm. Nestlé's condensed milk, La Lechera, or chocolate syrup were available to be poured on top. To prepare nachos, a yellowy cheese sauce from a 3 liter plastic bag was placed in a bowl and heated in the microwave. Two minutes later, the plastic-like cheese became liquid, ready to be poured over the portions of packaged corn-chips served in small foam bowls. Both the hot cakes and the nachos were prepared in a few minutes. Peeling off and slicing fruits took longer.

The convenience and profitability of these ultra-processed products contrasted with the intense labor required for handmade foods. In 2016, *tostadas, empanadas* and *picadas*—or *antojitos*, as people in the state of Veracruz call these and other *masa*-based foods—featured on the school menu at least three times a week. Foods like soups and stews were also cooked, but to a lesser extent. The affinity of students and their families for *antojitos* has two possible explanations. The first one has a cultural dimension. Andrés, who had worked in the school for more than 10 years and lived in a nearby town, considered that "*antojitos* are a tradition, a deeply rooted eating habit". Equally, Angel, a male teacher in his mid-30s, commented that in his six years at Emiliano Zapata Primary School he had noticed a deep kinship for "*masa, empanadas, enchiladas, taquitos* or, in short, for *antojitos*". Beyond its cultural roots, however, the students' affinity for *antojitos* can also be explained, as Andrés contentiously remarked, by their energetic contribution to, or their utility in, students' diets. "If our little kids don't have *antojitos* with the basic ingredients—*masa, salsa*, cheese and *frijolitos*—during the school breakfast, they will be hungry and asking for food at noon".[16]

While Andrés associated the consumption of *antojitos* with an energetic function, he also considered that "*masa*-based foods, together with *salsas* and beans, are widely consumed by kids from poor families, because those are cheap ingredients". *Antojitos* are culturally significant, tasty food, but they are also a conveniently cheap meal. For this reason, some kids did not use the food service at the school and instead received homemade *antojitos* delivered at break time. Every day, for instance, I observed a mother who delivered *empanadas* to her three sons. She could not afford to pay 30 pesos for three school breakfasts. With the same amount of money, this mother preferred to buy 1kg of *masa*, one cooking oil bottle and 250 grams of *quesillo*, and make *empanadas* for the whole family for the day.

Masa is central to diets in Veracruz. Yet SUMA-Nutrir and the *Lineamientos* have worked to stigmatize foods that are primarily made from it. Emiliano Zapata Primary School was closely monitored during the implementation of these strategies. One of the central messages people in the school got from this policy and program was that cooking *masa*-based food too often was not the best for students' health. Due to their ingredients, *masa* and fats, and the frying method employed in their preparation, *antojitos* were considered 'unhealthy' and 'harmful' foods by health and education authorities and "experts". The relationship between the accessible price of *antojitos*, the nature of their ingredients and their energetic content, however, contested the energy balance discourse.

At the discursive level, as discussed in Chapter 3, this premise assumes that food, or "energy in", is already *there*, available for people to consume it. Therefore, under the simplistic energy balance equation, people can be held responsible for either not choosing the 'right' food or for not expending enough energy.

However, the affection for *antojitos* of the Emiliano Zapata Primary School students tells us that the kind of energy consumed is not always a "choice", but a *need* that, of course, is culturally and economically shaped.

The idea of healthy lifestyles, as I stated in Chapter 1, has positioned schools as ideal spaces to 'fight' obesity through promoting 'healthy' diets. In schools, however, on a day-to-day basis this idea takes shape in a chaotic context. Policies and programs promoting 'healthy' eating, for instance, imagine schools to be fully equipped and have the resources to provide food to children. They also talk about food in a technical language that reduces it to "energy" with just a biological function. The above stories challenge this view through a description of how food comes to exist in schools amidst scarceness, labor and politics. The politically motivated misuse of funding allocated to Emiliano Zapata Primary School hindered the staff's working capacities. Nonetheless, in their everyday engagements around food, the school community mobilized to overcome structural problems and to challenge the reductionist perspectives of food and health deployed by healthy lifestyles.

Feeding children in Emiliano Zapata Primary School was a collective effort. The production of food resulted from the interaction of the staff, who contributed in different forms. In this school, students had food from the kitchen even if they had not paid for the breakfast. This put more pressure on to the school finances. Money was always scarce, but the *will to serve*, as the cooks used to say, replaced it. Working in the kitchen required cooking skills, but also the ability to endure hard conditions and to care through cooking (Gaddis, 2020; Poppendieck, 2010).

Unlike Elena, who always wanted to convince me that she sold "healthy food", the four cooks never talked about food in any term associated to health. I can say that they were, instead, guided by an understanding of food from where cooking was seen as the process through which an expression of care materialized in an edible object. Knowing that ingredients were scarce, for example, the cooks at Emiliano Zapata Primary School cautiously used them in cooking, trying to make the most out of them. However, when it came to pleasing the students' stomachs, they never minded giving more than was stipulated, in the "rule" or the budget. Similarly, the cooks considered that handmaking complex, tasty foods way of expressing their care for the students. In the next section, I elaborate further on this point and discuss the competing roles food has in Mexican schools, and the impacts of this on policy.

Masa, Fats and Love: The Social Life of *Real* Food

One warm morning in May 2016, I was in Emiliano Zapata Primary School's kitchen chatting with the Doñitas as they were industriously preparing *tostadas.*[17] Beatriz was making *masa* cakes with her hands, flattening them with her palm and placing the flattened *masa* on the griddle. After 20–30 seconds, the half-cooked flattened *masa* started to become a tortilla. At this point, Moni turned the tortillas over and cooked them for about the same time. Once the tortillas puffed up, Moni took them off the griddle and handed them to Angela, who began to poke the tortillas with a toothpick. Intrigued by this unknown technique, I asked why they made the holes. "If we don't puncture the tortillas, they absorb more oil when they're fried", Angela answered, placing the tortilla she had just punctured on the table. Doña Martha was sautéing garlic and onion in a bit of lard to fry the *frijolitos*.[18] I offered to help. Drying the sweat dripping from her face with her apron, Doña Martha chortled, "You don't know how to *tortear*. Men never cook".[19]

Rafa, the multi-purpose janitor, arrived with a big bunch of cilantro, two 500 mL cans of cream and a 3 kg bag of brown sugar. Visibly shattered, Rafa unscrewed her bottle of *Coca*, as Coca-Cola is commonly known in Mexico, and had a couple of gulps. "That's the last time that I go to the *tiendita*! It's too hot", she said. I checked the weather in my phone: it felt like 36 °C at 9:10 am. After cooling down, Rafa opened the sugar bag and dropped the whole bag into the 50 L pot used to prepare fresh fruit water. She then blended the cilantro with tomatoes, onion, garlic and jalapeño chilies to make a *salsa*.

Subtly, using no more than a gesture and the authority in her gaze, Doña Martha directed Angela to fry the tortillas. Angela first organized the punctured tortillas in pairs, then threw a piece of *masa* into the large, shallow metal frying pan of oil. Bubbles rose around the small piece of *masa*, which meant the oil temperature was right. Angela submerged the first two tortillas, spreading oil around them with a slotted metal spoon. Less than a minute later, she removed the deep-fried tortillas from the frying pan and stood them vertically over a metal bowl with holes at the bottom. The fried tortillas, the *frijolitos* and the *salsa* were ready. These ingredients plus chopped lettuce and cream were then assembled to create one of the students' favorite foods: *tostadas*.

Food in Benito Juárez and Emiliano Zapata primary schools was much more than nutrients. The practices of cooking, selling and eating food I observed were shaped by the local economic conditions and culture. The provisioning of food to students was more "business-oriented" in the former and more "cooperative" within the latter. Size mattered. Feeding 140 students is not the same as feeding nearly 1,000 students. Yet there were also general similarities between how food was made, sold and consumed within them. Notably, the production and sale of food was a source of income for both Benito Juárez and Emiliano Zapata primary schools and for their communities. Another similarity was that, while a variety of products were on offer, *real food* was central in both schools.

My emphasis on *real*, following Scrinis (2013), is intended to distinguish food that goes through a social process—like the *tostadas* in the above story—from industrial edible products—the ultra-processed products that I have alluded to throughout this book—that are mass-produced in factories from ingredients that one is barely aware of. Through this distinction I aim to offer a counternarrative to the policy construction of cooking and the provisioning of food in school as mere technical procedures.

In policy documents, as Chapter 3 showed, school cooks are depicted as depoliticized, mostly passive subjects who lack the skills required to prepare 'healthy' food. Yet the stories in this chapter have argued otherwise. School cooks are owners of contextual culinary knowledges that enable them to resourcefully over-come any difficulty in the kitchen. They care for the students in their own terms. They do so through the cultural practice of *cooking*. Doña Martha, Beatriz, Moni and Angela, for instance, knew perfectly that students loved *masa*-based foods and they prided themselves on satisfying this desire. Paradoxically, while all the school foods were made from scratch and involved hard work, the preparation of *antojitos* demanded even more. For the Doñitas, this posed no problem. Indeed, they happily engaged in the production of labor-intense *masa*-foods because cooking what students liked was—they proudly claimed—their form of expressing *love* and care.

This chapter has explained how food becomes to exist in schools amidst local tensions, macroeconomic change, power dynamics and the scarceness of resources. Its intention was to provide a from-the-ground critique to the reductionist per-spective on food implicit in policy. It has also shown an alternative story to the dominant narrative which presents schools both as part of the obesity problem and *the* solution to it. My emphasis on cooking aims to bring the reader's attention to an often-relegated point in school food regulations: the fact that food is socially, politically and economically produced. I will finish this chapter detailing how the practices of thinking and acting about food and health that are put forward through 'healthy lifestyles' are contested in the day-to-day cooking in Emiliano Zapata Primary School.

On an extremely hot May day around noon, I was in the dining area writing my notes. Inside the kitchen, conversations and cleaning noises could be heard while music played loudly on the radio. The Doñitas were hurriedly washing the dishes, mopping the floor and putting the few leftovers in containers to be taken home. Doña Martha came out to sweep the dining room. "It's very hot", I said. "It is!", she exclaimed. Building upon previous conversations, I said, "So, you have been part of the school for a long time". "Yes. I like to serve. I like to contribute and work for the community", Doña Martha uttered, wiping the sweat from her forehead. "Also, my sons are married, and my husband is always working. So, I come here, do something productive, have some food and receive 80 pesos. I enjoy it. I like to help. I like to cook". I confessed my fondness for her tasty food. "It's because I *cook with love*. Love is the secret ingredient that even if you eat only *frijolitos*, they will be tasty because of the love!", Doña Martha stated proudly.

The idea that "food is love" may be a cliché for many (see Roberts, 2015). If taken as a discourse, "food is love" has been mobilized for different purposes. Marketing to increase the consumption of ultra-processed products is doubtless a good example (see Antúnez et al., 2021). Food is love is a fixed statement. Under the conditions experienced in Santa Rosa, the food-is-love association can also make deep socio-economic inequalities. When Doña Martha stated that "even if you eat only *frijolitos*, they will be tasty because of the love", she was implicitly expressing how the combination of dreadfully low salaries and the rise in food prices (Avalos, 2016; Wood et al., 2012) made the worse off even more depen-dent on a few particular foods. While *frijolitos* have been part of the Mexican diet even from before the colonial era, and most Mexicans appreciate them, their consumption has also been constructed as a class distinction: beans are associated with poverty (Lutz & Miranda Mora, 2018; Ochoa Rivera, 2013).[20]

However, I think it can be fruitful to explore the idea of *food as love*, which, I suggest, is what Doña Martha was talking about. In the context of cooking, love can mean different things to people in different geographical locations; for some, this association might be meaningless. As a Mexican who was raised by a working-class, deeply catholic granny who treasured giving love through food, I interpret Doña Martha's meaning of love as the devotion invested in transforming dispersed, many times scarce, ingredients into a flavorful meal that fulfils not only the stomach but also the soul. This love, however, was not only verbal; it was also made material in the day-to-day practices of cooking.[21]

Doña Martha managed the school kitchen as if she were administering her own household: resourcefully, patiently and generously. Knowing that ingredients were scarce, she cautiously used them in cooking. While mentoring the other women in the art of cooking, she was tough, but loving. Above all, Doña Martha, as a Mexican working-class grandma, administered the kitchen not only with the aim of providing food, but also with the ultimate purpose of caring and expressing *love* through food. Perhaps this romantic interpretation of Doña Martha is nothing more than the result of my own biases. I accept this critique. Inexorably, as I problematized in Chapter 1, seeing Doña Martha in action led me back to my own childhood, reminiscing about Conchita. However, what I want to highlight through this narrative is that the neoliberal form of government has not completely transformed cultural dynamics.

The neoliberal policies that have been enacted since the 1980s have transformed Mexico politically and economically. But they have not been entirely successful in disseminating the "enterprise form" that, as Foucault (2008) claims, is fundamental for the success and maintenance of neoliberal governmentality. This

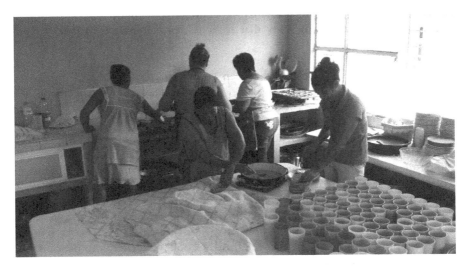

Figure 5.3 Cooking *real* food in Emiliano Zapata Primary School. Photo by the author.

is why, as Claudia herself stated in our interview (Chapter 4), Nestlé has sought to eradicate the language that associates homemade food with grannies and love. "That's wrong", Claudia emphasized, justifying why Nestlé wanted to "change" the fact that "in Mexican culture, food is love". Nestlé sought to make Mexicans adopt a technical language that quantifies food in calories and portions. However, speaking of *food as love* is a discursive form of resistance against the nutritional reductionism implicit in 'healthy lifestyles'.

From this perspective, the love that Doña Martha spoke about was materialized in the passionate cooking practices performed in the kitchen. Love manifested in the cooks' own descriptions of how they overcame the tough working conditions they faced. "I think we have given our best... we care for the kids", Beatriz emphasized, when I asked what could be done for children to access 'healthier' food [*comida más saludable*] at school.[22] "We have given our best", Doña Martha seconded. "Many times, we even make miracles!". Every single day during my fieldwork, I witnessed miracles being achieved in the kitchen. There were never enough ingredients, but the cooks always made miracles:

BEATRIZ: A kid told me, "Wow! [¡A su mecha!], the stew was delicious, but it had very little, almost no meat! You should have given me a bit more meat!" (all laugh)
JOSÉ: Cooking meals with meat is quite hard...
DOÑA MARTHA: Yes... for 10 pesos... how much is a kilo [of meat]?
BEATRIZ: Chicken meat... what we do, we milk the chicken, perfectly shredding every piece.
DOÑA MARTHA: That's why we make miracles!
MONI: Some kids don't want meat, sometimes they only want *frijolitos*, or some kids don't like cheese... and we have to find the way to...
BEATRIZ: We try to find the way to feed the kids! We don't like them to go without food, so we are always trying to devise something...
DOÑA MARTHA: That's why I say that *we're always doing miracles* [her and my emphasis]!

The quasi-religious association between food scarcity, sacrifice and care epitomizes the refusal of a bio-political project that, using discursive arrangements and practices, has tried to make Mexicans subjects of a neoliberal regime of health and living. Nonetheless, the lines of the *dispositif* that are working to subject these women and their cooking practices to a discursive construction of a rational decision maker have not found anchorage points. One explanation for this, though simplistic, would be that schools like Emiliano Zapata Primary School, and its community, lack so many resources that simply telling them to eat 'healthy' food merely becomes empty words that are forgotten as soon as they are uttered. However, with this idea I am diminishing both the agency of the various actors and the possible positive contributions that food strategies can have in schools. Therefore, I prefer to stand by the idea that the cooks integrated into their practice something from the myriad programs they have been exposed to. But they did so by adapting them to their own needs and for the students' benefit.

In their cooking, the cooks resisted the normative, technical character of 'healthy lifestyles', and instead continued to be guided by a view of food as a form of caring. The cooks never spoke of food in terms of biological 'health' qualities. Doña Martha only used *saludable* to describe food once, and that was after I put that word in her mouth. Nonetheless, in their own way, the cooks were also conscious of the adverse effects that frequent, high consumption of vegetable oil represents for human health.[23] They knew that offering *empanadas* too often was not ideal, because they were deep-fried. Yet they did not hesitate in adding a bit of lard to the griddle to give food "more flavor!", as they enthusiastically stated.

Across obesity and healthy eating policies food has been constructed as a strictly biological object which can be measured, quantified and restricted. These healthy lifestyles strategies have equally reduced cooking to a technical procedure, detaching this process from its cultural and historical roots. In the school-based healthy eating policies I discuss in this book, it is assumed that schools have the means to feed students. Yet the processes that occur before a student can put food in their mouth are absent. The detailed descriptions of how food becomes to exist, and how it is consumed, within Emiliano Zapata and Benito Juárez primary schools are intended to bring to attention the commonly neglected social dimension of food and cooking.

Future policy aimed at changing food practices in schools needs to move beyond the technical and reductionist view of food and be closer to the language used by mothers cooking in schools. The cooks in Emiliano Zapata and Benito Juárez primary schools do not lack the skills to prepare 'healthy' food; they are the owners of extensive practical knowledge about what and how to cook to sate hungry stomachs, most of the times under a tight budget and adverse conditions. Similarly, mothers and students do not lack the knowledge to take healthy food choices; what they lack on many occasions is *time* and economic resources. Small, but important, manifestations of resistance like the ones described in this chapter express the lack of viability of a bio-political project that, in reducing food to a measurable object, tries to disseminate an understanding on health and life that shares its foundations with a neoliberal form of government.

Conclusion

Through the ethnographic-inspired data discussed in this chapter, I illustrated how healthy lifestyles came to frame, or be rejected in, the day-to-day food practices of Benito Juárez and Emiliano Zapata primary schools. I have emphasized that context matters. The implementation of any school-based policy or program is adopted, contested or ignored depending on the particular political, economic and cultural conditions surrounding a school. Therefore, this chapter is also an empirical response to the discursive construction of schools as 'anti-obesity' sites. Through these data, I seek to broaden the space for critical conversations in obesity policymaking.

It is beyond my intention to judge the accuracy or moral implications of the actions taken in the schools to encourage students to lead healthier lives. Nor have

I intended to evaluate policy. I have purposefully highlighted the differences between the two schools to show the diversity of ideas about the relationship between food and health, the role of schools in 'fighting' obesity and the place of food in schools. I also ruled out obesity as a topic of the discussion, to be consistent with my idea of telling a different story about this issue.

Another important point raised was that the provision of food, as almost any activity in public schools, is done amidst insufficient resources. As has been described in earlier sections, political corruption has motivated the misuse of education funding. For this reason, principals and teachers have to find channels to access the resources required for schools. This was the case in both schools. The infrastructure and the human resources in both Emiliano Zapata and Benito Juárez primary schools were more the outcome of "personal connections", than the result of government support.[24]

While in some cases school community members were imbued by the 'healthy lifestyles' language, this chapter has also shown how others escaped from the lines that attempt to make them 'healthy' subjects. Through different strategies, teachers, students, parents and cooks have challenged the discourses and discursive practices seeking to make them rational, self-responsible subjects who individualistically care for their health. No one captures the essence of this resistance better than the Doñitas in the kitchen at Emiliano Zapata Primary School. I have decided to be optimistic, perhaps at the risk of being labelled as too romantic, in my concluding discussions of the data. To break the *dispositif*, I have come to understand, one needs to find points where resistance can be anchored. For this reason, I have borrowed the language and optimism used by the cooks, in spite of the hardships they face. Making these voices heard can start shifting the dominant discourse.

However, I will now move to present a less optimistic point. In the next chapter I demonstrate that, although it has faced resistance, the *dispositif of healthy lifestyles* has been working to aid the interests of corporations.

Notes

1 A literal translation of "Jornadas de Cierre" would be "Wrap-up Sessions". According to Victoria and Claudia, these events revealed that mothers "needed" more ideas about "how to cook healthy food". Therefore, in the 2012–2013 school year a call for "local recipes from Veracruz" was launched across the DEPE. The winning recipes would become part of a cookbook that would be edited, printed and distributed between the DEPE and Nestlé. For details on the politics of production of this cookbook, and other materials, see Chapter 4.

2 Bakić Hayden (2014), Long-Solís (2007) and Roever (2010) have shown that neoliberal policies have considerably increased the size of the informal economy, making many people reliant on street food selling. Beyond my culinary chauvinism, I see what today is called "Mexican food" as the result of centuries of cultural transformations, global trade, political decisions and struggles over meaning. For excellent examples on these issues, see Aguilar-Rodríguez (2007, 2009, 2011); Bak-Geller Corona (2009, 2013); Ochoa (2002); and Pilcher (1998, 2004, 2013).

3 I will elaborate more on this point in the conclusion of this chapter and in the final chapter of the book.

4 My approach to food is influenced by Appadurai (1981), Mintz (1985) and Scrinis (2013). For an elaboration on my treatment of school food, see Tenorio (2022).

5 Elsie Rockwell's (1994, 2009) anthropological approach to the study of schools and schooling practices has significantly influenced my development of this chapter.

6 See note 17 in Chapter 1.

7 According to a report from SEP and OECD (2013), on average, principals in Mexico obtain this leadership position at the age of 52, after having worked for 24 years as generalist teachers.

8 Double-shift schools are common in Mexico. According to Bray (2008), these kinds of schools usually operate in poor countries to relieve financial pressures and minimise costs. If Benito Juárez Primary School was not a "double-shift school", another school would need to be constructed in Paso de Leones to cover all the children in the catchment. Only the principal, two curriculum advisers and a couple of teachers worked both the two shifts. The rest worked only in the morning shift. Teachers working two shifts are paid double.

9 The LISTO Diploma was the developed by Worldfund, now called 'Educando'. As a report from Educando (2018, p. 23) states, LISTO aims to provide "training and support through coaching for school leaders to directly transform school culture, with the goal of improving the quality of education and learning". Worldfund was created in 2002 by Luanne Zurlo. As the organisation's website states, Zurlo "left Goldman Sachs and a successful nine-year career on Wall Street to start Educando (founded as World Education & Development Fund – Worldfund)" after a trip to Mexico where she "learned about the lack of quality education available for most Latin American children" (Educando, n.d.).

10 *Picadas*, or *picaditas*, are small tortillas with a lip formed around the edged, topped with beans, green or red salsa, onion and cheese.

11 I am drawing this conclusion borrowing from the sociology of education literature that has extensively reported on the various ways in which corporations and profit-driven organizations are shaping education policy and practice globally. For examples, see Ball (2009), Hogan (2016), Hogan et al. (2016), Macdonald, Johnson & Lingard (2020).

12 I have used a feminine name to maintain the town's anonymity and to acknowledge that, although they played a central role, women's participation in the Mexican Revolution is hardly mentioned in the literature. For the participation of women in the revolution, see Fowler-Salamini (2013) and Fowler-Salamini and Vaughan (1994). Fowler-Salamini (1970, 1978) and Ginzberg (1997, 1998, 2000) have thoroughly analyzed the agrarian movement in Veracruz between 1920 and 1938. The name changes for Santa Rosa and other cities in Mexico can be found in INEGI's (n.d.) online database. Carmen Serdán was not part of Veracruz League of Agrarian Communities. She was an important organizer of the revolution movement in the state of Puebla.

13 For a detailed report, see Auditoría Superior de la Federación (2013).

14 Pike (2008) discusses how the spatial arrangements in school dining rooms shape the eating practices of students. Through a "governmentality" lens, Pike suggests that the spatial disposition of dining rooms in schools in the United Kingdom works to "normalize" children's engagements with food.

15 Before NAFTA, Veracruz used to attract migrants from nearby states.

16 Multiple forms of *masa* and fats of different kinds have been central ingredients in Mexican's day-to-day cooking and eating practices. A study of food consumption in 1970s' Mexico, for example, showed that products made out of *masa*, lard and vegetable oil were among the most-consumed food products among a large segment of the population (Lustig, 1980). However, amidst the 'fight' against obesity, the relevance of these ingredients in Mexican diets has become contentious (see García-García et al., 2008; Treviño Ronzón & Sánchez Pacheco, 2014).

17 *Tostadas* are deep-fried tortillas topped with black beans, lettuce, cheese, cream, shredded chicken and sauce. On Emiliano Zapata Primary School's menu, only *tostadas* without chicken were available.
18 *Frijoles* mean beans in English. In Mexico, the suffix *ito/ita* is added to multiple words as a way to express a particular emphasis. The suffix *ito/ita* is widely added to food names. When used in foods, similar to *frijolitos* or *picaditas*, it usually denotes the appreciation for the time and effort that has been put into cooking and the emotional value assigned to food.
19 *Tortear* is the verb used for the action of shaping *masa* with the palm of one's hand to prepare different *masa*-based foods like tortillas, *empanadas, picaditas* or *gorditas*.
20 For a more optimistic, less class-centered, interpretation of bean consumption in Mexico, see Amerlinck (2012).
21 Abarca's (2006) book *Voices in the Kitchen* discusses how working-class Mexican and Mexican-American women portray their worldviews through cooking, and the central role the kitchen has in the making of these women.
22 I am using inverted commas around healthier to highlight the reductionism implicit in my own question, which is denoted in my use of the word *saludable* but also in the way I assumed that *masa*-based foods were not as 'healthy' as other foods could be. Through a close reading of my interview transcripts, I noticed that it was me who spoke of food in technical terms, which sometimes influenced the answers of my interviewees.
23 The consumption of vegetable oil, a form of fat, has increased steadily since the 1950s. In a country where a large section of the population used lard in food preparation, advertising played a central role to transform this practice, particularly through pushing the idea that vegetable oil was a 'healthier' option—a fact which is still debatable (see Scrinis, 2013; Willet, 1994)—and a product that was "classier" than lard (Aguilar-Rodríguez, 2009). From the mid-1990s, the agribusiness transformations introduced by NAFTA have also helped to increase the availability and consumption in Mexico of vegetable oil produced in the United States (Torres-Torres and Aguilar-Ortega, 2003; Yunez-Naude and Barceinas, 2002). However, in spite of these changes, the use of lard has remained a common practice among cooks to potentiate flavours.
24 Drawing on a broader understanding of what "corruption" means, Akhil Gupta (2012) claims that "low-level corruption" can help to ameliorate the state's inability to secure welfare and aid for particular sectors of the population. The principal of Emiliano Zapata Primary School at the time of my research, Andrés, occupied a high-level position at the state level of the Teachers' Union between 2007 and 2013. Like Susana and Rosalba, he also used his personal connections to gain favours for the school, which may be considered "corruption". However, with Gupta in mind, I prefer to say that doing this was the only way in which Emiliano Zapata Primary School could access much-needed resources.

References

Abarca, M. E. (2006). *Voices in the kitchen: Views of food and the world from working-class Mexican and Mexican American women*. Texas A&M University Press.
Aguilar-Rodríguez, S. (2007). Cooking modernity: Nutrition policies, class, and gender in 1940s and 1950s Mexico. *The Americas*, 64(2), 177–205. https://doi.org/10.1353/tam.2007.0128.
Aguilar-Rodríguez, S. (2009). La mesa está servida: Comida y vida cotidiana en el México de mediados del siglo XX [The table is served: Food and daily life in mid-twentieth century Mexico]. *HIB: Revista de Historia Iberoamericana*, 2(2), 52–85.
Aguilar-Rodríguez, S. (2011). Nutrition and modernity: Milk consumption in 1940s and 1950s Mexico. *Radical History Review* (110), 36–59. https://doi.org/10.1215/01636545-2010-025.

Amerlinck, M.-J. (2012). Rice and beans, a staple on even the most respectable Mexican tables. In R. Wilk & L. Barbosa (eds.), *Rice and beans: A unique dish in a hundred* (pp. 219–240). Berg.

Antúnez, L., Alcaire, F., Brunet, G., Bove, I., & Ares, G. (2021). COVID-washing of ultra-processed products: the content of digital marketing on Facebook during the COVID-19 pandemic in Uruguay. *Public Health Nutrition*, 24(5), 1142–1152. https://doi.org/10.1017/S1368980021000306.

Appadurai, A. (1981). Gastro-politics in Hindu South Asia. *American Ethnologist*, 8(3), 494–511. http://www.jstor.org/stable/644298.

Auditoría Superior de la Federación (2013). *Programa de Escuelas de Tiempo Completo (PETC)* [*Full-time scheme schools program (PETC)*]. https://www.asf.gob.mx/Trans/Informes/IR2013i/Documentos/Auditorias/2013_MR-ESCUELAS%20DE%20TIEMPO%20COMPLETO_a.pdf.

Avalos, A. (2016). Household consumption response to food price shocks and the vulnerability of the poor in Mexico. *Journal of International Development*, 28(8), 1294–1312. https://doi.org/10.1002/jid.3127.

Bak-Geller Corona, S. (2009). Los recetarios "afrencesados" del siglo XIX en México. La construcción de la nación mexicana y de un modelo culinario nacional [French-fashioned Mexican recipe books in the 19th century. Globalization and construction of a national culinary model]. *Anthropology of Food*, S6(I). https://doi.org/10.4000/aof.6464.

Bak-Geller Corona, S. (2013). Narrativas deleitosas de la nación. Los primeros libros de cocina en México (1830–1890) [Narratives of nation-making. The first cookbooks in Mexico (1830–1890)]. *Desacatos*, 43(September–December), 31–44.

Bakić Hayden, T. (2014). The taste of precarity: Language, legitimacy, and legality among Mexican street food vendors. In R. D. C. Vieira Cardoso, M. Companion, & S. R. Marras (eds.), *Street food: Culture, economy, health and governance* (pp. 83–98). Routledge.

Ball, S. J. (2009). Privatising education, privatising education policy, privatising educational research: Network governance and the 'competition state'. *Journal of Education Policy*, 24(1), 83–99. https://doi.org/10.1080/02680930802419474.

Bray, M. (2008). *Double-shift schooling: design and operation for cost-effectiveness*. Fundamentals of Education Planning. http://unesdoc.unesco.org/images/0016/001636/163606e.pdf.

Educando (2018). Educando by WorldFund: Inspiring teachers, creating leaders, transforming lives. https://educando.org.

Educando (n.d.). Our story. https://educando.org/our-story/.

Foucault, M. (2008). *The birth of biopolitics: Lectures at the Collège De France 1978–1979*, translated by G. Burchell. Picador.

Fowler-Salamini, H. (1970). Orígenes Laborales de la Organización Campesina en Veracruz [Labour origins of the Peasant Organization in Veracruz]. *Historia Mexicana*, 20(2), 235–264. https://historiamexicana.colmex.mx/index.php/RHM/article/view/2508/2020.

Fowler-Salamini, H. (1978). *Agrarian radicalism in Veracruz, 1920–38*. University of Nebraska Press.

Fowler-Salamini, H. (2013). *Working women, entrepreneurs and the Mexican Revolution: The coffee culture of Córdoba, Veracruz*. University of Nebraska Press.

Fowler-Salamini, H., & Vaughan, M. K. (1994). *Women of the Mexican countryside, 1850–1990: Creating spaces, shaping transitions*. University of Arizona Press.

Gaddis, J. E. (2020). *The labor of lunch: Why we need real food and real jobs in American public schools*. University of California Press.

García-García, E., De la Lata-Romero, M., Kaufer-Horwitz, M., Tusié-Luna, M. T., Calzada-León, R., Vázquez-Velázquez, V., ... Sotelo-Morales, J. (2008). La obesidad y el síndrome metabólico como problema de salud pública. Una reflexión [Obesity and metabolic syndrome as public health problems. A reflection]. *Salud Pública de México*, 50(6), 530–547.

Ginzberg, E. (1997). Ideología, política y la cuestión de las prioridades: Lázaro Cárdenas y Adalberto Tejeda, 1928–1934 [Politics, ideology and priorities: Lázaro Cárdenas and Adalberto Tejeda, 1928–1934]. *Mexican Studies/Estudios Mexicanos*, 13(1), 55–85. https://doi.org/10.2307/1051866.

Ginzberg, E. (1998). State agrarianism versus democratic agrarianism: Adalberto Tejeda's experiment in Veracruz, 1928–32. *Journal of Latin American Studies*, 30(2), 341–372. https://doi.org/10.1017/S0022216X98005070.

Ginzberg, E. (2000). Formación de la infraestructura política para una reforma agraria radical: Adalberto Tejeda y la cuestión municipal en Veracruz, 1928–1932 [Laying the political ground for a radical agrarian reform: Adalberto Tejeda's uses of municipality in Veracruz, 1928–2923]. *Historia Mexicana*, 49(4), 673–727.

Gupta, A. (2012). *Red tape: Bureaucracy, structural violence and poverty in India*. Duke University Press.

Hogan, A. (2016). NAPLAN and the role of edu-business: New governance, new privatisations and new partnerships in Australian education policy. *The Australian Educational Researcher*, 43(1), 93–110. https://doi.org/10.1007/s13384-014-0162-z.

Hogan, A., Sellar, S., & Lingard, B. (2016). Commercialising comparison: Pearson puts the TLC in soft capitalism. *Journal of Education Policy*, 31(3), 243–258. https://doi.org/10.1080/02680939.2015.1112922.

INEGI (n.d.). Archivo histórico de localidades geoestadísticas [Archive of locations and geo-statistics]. https://www.inegi.org.mx/app/geo2/ahl/#.

Levine, S. (2008). *School lunch politics: The surprising history of America's favorite welfare program*. Princeton University Press.

Lineamientos 2010 (Acuerdo mediante el cual se establecen los lineamientos generales para el expendio o distribución de alimentos y bebidas en los establecimientos de consumo escolar de los planteles de educación básica [General guidelines for the distribution or sales of food and drinks by retailers within basic education schools]) (2010). Diario Oficial de la Federación: Órgano del Gobierno Constitucional de los Estados Unidos Mexicanos.

Lineamientos 2014 (Acuerdo mediante el cual se establecen los lineamientos generales para el expendio y distribución de alimentos y bebidas preparados y procesados en las escuelas del Sistema Educativo Nacional [Guidelines for the sales and distribution of prepared and processed food and drinks in the Mexican national education system]) (2014). Diario Oficial de la Federación: Órgano del Gobierno Constitucional de los Estados Unidos Mexicanos.

Long-Solís, J. (2007). A survey of street foods in Mexico City. *Food and Foodways*, 15(3–4), 213–236. https://doi.org/10.1080/07409710701620136.

Lustig, N. (1980). Distribución del ingreso y consumo de alimentos en México [Income distribution and food consumption in Mexico]. *Demografía y economía*, 14(2), 214–245. http://www.jstor.org/stable/40602232.

Lutz, B., & Miranda Mora, M. S. (2018). El bien comer: Normalización de las prácticas alimentarias en México [Good eating: Standardization of food practices in Mexico]. *Iberoforum. Revista de Ciencias Sociales de la Universidad Iberoamericana*, 13(26), 72–97.

Macdonald, D., Johnson, R., & Lingard, B. (2020). Globalisation, neoliberalisation, and network governance: An international study of outsourcing in health and physical education. *Discourse: Studies in the Cultural Politics of Education*, 41(2), 169–186. https://doi.org/10.1080/01596306.2020.1722422.

Mintz, S. W. (1985). *Sweetness and power: The place of sugar in modern history*. Penguin Books.

Ochoa, E. (2002). *Feeding Mexico: The political use of food since 1910*. Scholarly Resources Inc.

Ochoa Rivera, T. (2013). Alimentacióny diferenciación social: El caso de una comunidad en México [Food and social differentiation: The case of a community in Mexico]. *Revista Internacional de Ciencias Sociales*, 2(1), 9–20. https://doi.org/10.37467/gka-revsocial.v2.1227.

Pike, J. (2008). Foucault, space and primary school dining rooms. *Children's Geographies*, 6 (4), 413–422. https://doi.org/10.1080/14733280802338114.

Pilcher, J. M. (1998). *Que vivan los tamales! Food and the making of Mexican identity*. University of New Mexico Press.

Pilcher, J. M. (2004). Industrial tortillas and folkloric Pepsi: The nutritional consequences of hybrid cuisines in Mexico. In J. L. Watson & M. L. Caldwell (eds.), *The cultural politics of food and eating: A reader* (pp. 235–250). Wiley-Blackwell.

Pilcher, J. M. (2013). Taco Bell, Maseca, and Slow Food: A postmodern apocalypse for Mexico's peasant cuisine? In C. Counihan & P. Van Esterik (eds.), *Food and culture: A reader* (3rd ed., pp. 426–436). Routledge.

Poppendieck, J. (2010). *Free for all: Fixing school food in America*. University of California Press.

Roberts, E. F. S. (2015). Food is love: And so, what then? *BioSocieties*, 10(2), 247–252. https://doi.org/10.1057/biosoc.2015.18.

Rockwell, E. (1994). Schools of the revolution: Enacting and contesting state forms in Tlaxcala, 1910–1030. In G. M. Joseph & D. Nugent (eds.), *Everyday forms of state formation. Revolution and the negotiation of rule in modern Mexico* (pp. 170–208). Duke University Press.

Rockwell, E. (2009). *La experiencia etnográfica: Historia y cultura en los procesos educativos* [*The ethnographic experience: History and culture in educational processes*]. Paidós.

Roever, S. (2010). Street trade in Latin America: Demographic trends, legal issues and vending organisations in six cities. In S. Bhowmik (ed.), *Street vendors in the global urban economy* (pp. 208–241). Routledge.

Scrinis, G. (2013). *Nutritionism: The science and politics of dietary advice*. Columbia University Press.

SEP & OCDE (2013). *México: Principales hallazgos del Estuido Internarional sobre la Enseñanza y el Aprendizaje (TALIS)* [*Mexico: Main findings from the Teaching and Learning International Survey*]. http://www.dgep.sep.gob.mx/BROW-AES/Talis/imagenes/NotaPais_Mexico_espa%C3%B1ol.pdf.

Tenorio, J. (2022). Encountering 'healthy' food in Mexican schools. In M. Gard, D. Powell, & J. Tenorio (eds.), *Routledge handbook of critical obesity studies* (pp. 144–153). Routledge.

Torres-Torres, F., & Aguilar-Ortega, T. (2003). Aspectos externos de la vulnerabilidad alimentaria de México [External negative aspects on food security in Mexico]. In F. Torres-Torres (ed.), *Seguridad alimentaria: Seguridad nacional* (pp. 87–123). UNAM, Plaza y Valdés.

Treviño Ronzón, E., & Sánchez Pacheco, G. (2014). La Implementación de los Lineamientos para Regular el Expendio de Alimentos y Bebidas en dos Escuelas Telesecundarias de Veracruz. Análisis desde la Perspectiva de los Sujetos [The implementation of the Guidelines to Regulate Food and Drinks Sales in two secondary schools in Veracruz: The perspective of the participants]. *CPU-e: Revista de Investigación Educativa*, 19 (July–December), 60–85.

Willet, W. C. (1994). Diet and health: What should we eat? *Science*, 264(5158), 532–537. https://doi.org/10.1126/science.8160011.

Wood, B. D. K., Nelson, C. H., & Nogueira, L. (2012). Poverty effects of food price escalation: The importance of substitution effects in Mexican households. *Food Policy*, 37(1), 77–85. https://doi.org/10.1016/j.foodpol.2011.11.005.

Yunez-Naude, A., & Barceinas, F. (2002). *Lessons from NAFTA: The case of Mexico's agricultural sector*. Final Report to the World Bank. https://citeseerx.ist.psu.edu/document?repid=rep1&type=pdf&doi=85cdb8ada9ea5bfe53fd677f4b8507a17e666af9.

6 Healthy Lifestyles, Bottled Water and Corporate Profits

I visited Benito Juárez Primary School for the second time in the last week of April in 2016. I arrived at about 8:40 in a humid spring morning. I sat at one of the concrete benches facing the rear patio. In front of me, a group of first-grade students were finishing their physical education class. Carlos, a short student, left the group and approached me. "Hello", he said. "Hello", I replied. Surprised by the size of his backpack, I asked what he was carrying. "My supplies: books, a bottle of water, and", the seven-year-old said with proud emphasis, "my *whole-grain* sandwich".[1] Carlos asked who I was and what was I doing in the school. "I'm José, and I'm here to see what kids eat in the school and why", I said. My answer to his questions framed our conversation. We chatted for no more than three minutes. In this time, Carlos told me what he normally ate and drank at school, and at home. Carlos emphasized his fondness for *refrescos*, which is how carbonated sugary drinks are known in central and southern Mexico. "Before coming to school in the mornings", he said cheerfully, "that's what I drink—[a] *refresco*". Testing the nutritional literacy of this spirited kid, I asked what was better, water or *refrescos*. "Water!", responded Carlos straightaway. "But I prefer [a] *refresco* because it has lots of sugar, and *I love sugar!*".

During my days in Benito Juárez Primary School, I observed that Carlos generally drank water from a 1 L bottle of Ciel, Coca-Cola's water brand in Mexico. Like him, other students usually brought water bottles of Ciel; Epura, PepsiCo's brand; Bonafont, Danone's widely sold brand; or Sta.María, Nestlé's water in Mexico. The students also had the option to *buy* water in the school. Nutrilandia sold 600 mL-Ciel-bottles for 10 pesos. For the same price, students could get a 1 L bottle of any brand at nearby small, corner stores [*tienditas*] and at OXXOs, a chain of convenience stores (see Chapter 1). No more than a third of students regularly bought water from Nutrilandia. Most of them used to bring bottled water from outside school, either in single-use bottles bought nearby or in reusable bottles filled at home.

The *Lineamientos 2010* facilitated the consumption of water as the only hydration option in schools. Before this policy was released, sugary drinks of all sorts—notably *refrescos*—were widely available in schools. By 2016 the consumption of *refrescos* during the school time had been nearly eradicated in some schools. This was the case in Emiliano Zapata and Benito Juárez primary schools, at least while I was there. The *Lineamientos 2010*, however, did not achieve this goal on its own.

DOI: 10.4324/9781003356264-6

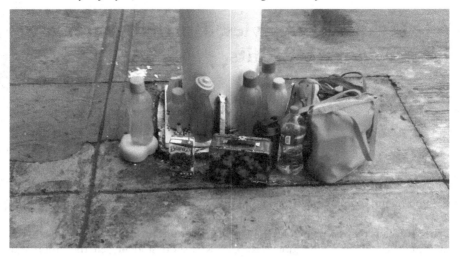

Figure 6.1 Bottles with water in Benito Juárez Primary School. Photo by the author.

The message that water is the healthier hydration option and that *refrescos* are bad for health was also reinforced through the work of teachers in the classroom. The implementation of healthy lifestyles programs like SUMA-Nutrir also aided to increase awareness among students of the dangers drinking *refrescos* posed to health. Evidence of the effectiveness of this message is the fact that Carlos, like most of the students, only drank water while at Benito Juárez Primary School.

The nearly complete eradication of the consumption of *refrescos* in some schools is undoubtedly one of the main achievements of healthy lifestyles. The fact that children recognize, as Carlos did, that drinking water is better than drinking *refrescos* is a significant public health triumph, which shows the extent to which consumer behavior can be, partially, modelled through the synergy of various policy actions. Yet the extent to which students' preference for *refrescos* has been eliminated can be questioned. Like Carlos, all the students I chatted with during my fieldwork distinguished between "good" and "bad" foods and "good" and "bad" drinks, and knew that the "bad foods" and "bad drinks"—like *refrescos*— should be avoided as much as possible. They knew that industrial snack foods were "junk", and drinking water should be preferred over consuming *refrescos*. Curiously, the children also emphasized their fondness for *refrescos* and claimed to be anxiously waiting to consume them outside the school (for similar evidence see Ortega-Avila et al., 2018).[2]

Healthy lifestyles, this book proposes, is a *dispositif,* or an ensemble of discourses, institutions, policies and practices that is working to govern the biological functions of the population. This *dispositif* has emerged in a context of market-driven economic reforms that have transformed the forms of living and consumption practices of the population and has enabled the dispersion of an "enterprise form", which is fundamental to the advancement of neoliberalism.

To frame this argument, Chapter 2 explained how the state in Mexico transited through phases of formation and transformations through the twentieth century, and how the transition from a nationalistic to an open-market economy enabled the conditions for healthy lifestyles to emerge as tool of government. Taking this historical context as background, Chapter 3 discussed the connection between economic reforms, change in public health policy and the corporate government of eating. Healthy lifestyles and its associated discourses, Chapter 3 showed, have come to be discursively assembled significantly by regimes of knowledge produced by market forces. One of the outstanding features of healthy lifestyles is that the interests of corporations are central to its workings. Chapter 4 described the implementation of a healthy lifestyles program, SUMA-Nutrir, between Secretaría de Educación de Veracruz (SEV) and Nestlé. My argument was that, through this program, Nestlé has disseminated its view on food and its relationship to health and increased its visibility among the population. Chapter 5 narrated stories of how food is made, sold, consumed and regulated in the everyday in schools. Its aim was to show how regulations came to be enmeshed with practices and material conditions, and how the imperative for being 'healthy' is challenged in the day-to-day practices of cooking in schools.

In this chapter, I discuss how the *dispositif of healthy lifestyles* has worked for the interests of food and drink corporations. Taking water consumption as my case for analysis, I show how the policies and programs launched to 'fight' obesity have been successful in, partially, halting the consumption of *refrescos* in schools, but at a cost. The fact that Mexican students, like Carlos, are drinking less *refrescos* inside schools should be celebrated, but it is equally important to say that this "success" has translated into profits for corporations.

The executive summary of the 2018 Soft Drinks in Mexico report by Euromonitor International (2018b, para. 1, emphasis added), for example, states that bottled water sales "observed interesting growth driven mostly by convenience and by the *adoption of healthier habits* by consumers". The report highlights that Mexicans were buying more bottled water because "they have been constantly reminded that drinking water is one of the most recommended habits to maintain their wellbeing".[3] This point was observably true in Benito Juárez and Emiliano Zapata primary schools. Students knew *refrescos* were not good for their health. They drank water within the school because they had no option. They nonetheless were lovers and regular consumers of *refrescos*, notably Coca-Cola, outside.

The consumption of water as the alternative to *refrescos* was also encouraged among the Mexican population through fiscal measures. In 2014, the Mexican government introduced a 1-peso-per-litre tax on sugary drinks—hereinafter referred to as sugar tax—with the aim of decreasing the consumption of these drinks. The sugar tax and the promotion of healthy lifestyles have aided to partially decrease the sale and consumption of *refrescos*. However, the sale of other types of sugary drinks such as industrial juices, teas, sport and energy drinks and flavored milks has been rising.[4] Furthermore, corporations created smaller presentations of their non-carbonated sugary drinks to comply with the technical nutritional details within the *Lineamientos*.

Changing the consumption of *refrescos* for water has not been easy, but the decisive work of teachers, as this chapter shows, and broader measures such as taxes have been partially successful in changing consumption behavior. Yet this change has also benefited other interests beyond public health. In Mexico tap water is not always good for human consumption and a stigma exists over drinking this water. One of the main public health arguments given by the proposers of the sugar tax was that tax revenue would be used to equip schools with the infrastructure needed to provide children with access to free, safe water. However, due to political corruption funds, unsurprisingly, never reached schools (see Auditoría Superior de la Federación, 2018). In this context, the promotion of water as the healthiest drink has created direct economic benefits for corporations.

In what follows, I describe how, from a historical point of view, tap water in Mexico came to be considered 'dangerous' for human consumption and how this widespread belief has facilitated the commodification of water in Mexico. Then, I discuss the science behind water consumption to show how, regardless of the lack of evidence, the constant consumption of water has been constructed as a health imperative by, in part, corporate forces. I also discuss the problems schools face in their day-to-day to provide water to students and the role teachers have had in making students drink less *refrescos*, at least within school hours. Finally, I empirically demonstrate the connection between the steady growth of bottled water sales and the promotion of healthy lifestyles in schools.

A Brief History of Bottled Water in Mexico

Regardless of their geographical location, gender, economic condition, employment and so forth, all the people who I talked to and interacted with during my fieldwork had one single thing in common. They only drank water from a *garrafón*, a 20 L bottle, or from plastic bottles in smaller sizes. Partly motivated by the wide-spread belief that tap water is "dangerous",[5] almost no one dared to drink water directly from the tap. In the schools, for example, cooking was done exclusively with garrafón water. Some students brought water in their reusable bottles, whereas others bought 600 mL bottles for 10 pesos at Nutrilandia, or for 6 pesos at Emiliano Zapata Primary School's principal's office.

On the streets, bottles of water from Coca-Cola, Nestlé, PepsiCo and Danone were everywhere. Inside OXXOs, bottles of water were stocked in fridges and others were conveniently located next to the counter. Bottled water sales, especially in small sizes ranging from 600 mL to 1.5 L, had surged in the 10 years leading up to my fieldwork (Barragán, 2015; Delgado-Ramos et al., 2014; Estrada-Vivas, 2016; Ortega Castañeda, 2016; Pacheco-Vega, 2015; Solís, 2017; Tourliere, 2015), mainly because of the discursive construction of water consumption as a synonym for health. However, Mexicans have been using water from garrafones, which technically are bottled water, to cook with and drink for a long time. In this section, I discuss how political decisions and a series of unexpected issues have pushed Mexicans to have limited access to tap water and to avoid its use. This background offers an explanation of how concrete conditions have facilitated the commodification of water, assisted by healthy lifestyles.

In the early twentieth century, water became one of the tools that the triumphant revolutionary groups used to strengthen the nascent Mexican state (Tortolero, 2000). Water resources were expropriated from private companies and transferred into state hands, with the aim of making them available for larger sectors of the population. Land ownership reforms in the 1930s enabled water springs to be partly protected from mass exploitation. Yet a constitutional change in 1994 enabled corporate access to these places. This privatization was aided by the fact that the distribution of water was trapped by politics and followed a clientelist logic rather than an "efficient, productive and environmentally safe perspective" (Aboites-Aguilar et al., 2010, p. 28). Until the late 1940s, the postrevolutionary Mexican state directed the funding for hydrological infrastructure, such as dams, to favor the agriculture and dairy sectors, with limited investment in other hydrological projects. Resources were channeled to extend the potable water and sewage networks into the nascent urban areas as industrial expansion took place. However, the process was slow. According to Aboites-Aguilar (2004), by 1970 only 61 percent of Mexican households had access to running water. The consumption of water directly from the tap was never common.

I did not find empirical sources that described when or why Mexicans started to drink water from garrafones. However, relatives and friends in Mexico told me that this practice has existed, at least in their experience, as early as the 1950s. Estrada-Vivas (2016) argues that the consumption of water from garrafones started to rise after 1985, amidst the chaos and disinformation generated after one of the strongest-recorded earthquakes struck Mexico City. Potable water and sewage infrastructure were heavily damaged, which created visible water contamination. Buying garrafones became common practice. After 1985 people in Mexico City developed "the belief that buying purified and bottled water was a matter of health" (Estrada-Vivas, 2016, p. 12).[6] Greene (2018) claims that this situation was aggravated in 1991, when a cholera outbreak erupted in Mexico. Although the Mexican government ran mass-media campaigns to encourage people to boil tap water or chlorinate it before consumption (Sepúlveda et al., 2006), Mexicans did not necessarily adopt these methods as part of their water-consumption practices. Instead, given that the market-friendly reforms of the late 1980s/early 1990s had facilitated the expansion and diversification of the bottled water market, Mexicans started to buy more water for their own consumption (Barragán, 2015; Delgado-Ramos et al., 2014; Lemus, 2019; Pacheco-Vega, 2015; Solís, 2017; Tourliere, 2015).

The earthquake in 1985 and the cholera outbreak in 1991 increased the consumption of garrafones. However, water in bottles of 600 mL, 1 L and 1.5 L sizes were still almost non-existent in the mid-1990s. These bottle sizes were introduced in the late 1990s or early 2000s, as Coca-Cola, PepsiCo, Danone and Nestlé entered a market which had previously been dominated by local companies. While the lack of hydrological infrastructure and the widespread distrust of tap water has made Mexicans consume water from bottles for a long time, I argue that the commodification of water has been powered by the *dispositif of healthy lifestyles* (for a similar point, see also Mazari-Hiriart et al., 2010). However, marketing and nutrition science around water consumption have also stimulated this phenomenon. Moreover, corporations with a stake in the water market significantly increased their funding of research on water after the 1990s. Together with the imperative for reducing energy intake as an 'anti-obesity' measure, scientific evidence was used to validate the idea that water needs to be drank plentifully and constantly. This is not bad. Yet an issue arises if the advice is given by a stakeholder with an economic interest in water. This problem also has implications in the commodification of water. If water needs to be drank constantly, but there is no public supply of safe drinkable water from the tap, people need to *buy* the water they consume.

The Uses of Water Consumption Science

I followed Carlos and the other First-Year students into their classroom. Lucia, the teacher, was sat at her desk marking. It was nearly 9 am. Lucia instructed the students to sit down and put their food for the *refrigerio* [a short snack break] over their desks. Following her instructions, I took out an apple from my bag. The little girl next to me exclaimed, "An apple!". "What did you bring?", I asked. "Nothing. Just water", the little girl replied, "because mum gave me money to buy *picaditas* and candies during the break". Carlos, who was sitting close by, chimed in: "I didn't bring money, but brought my whole-grain sandwich". He would eat half during the refrigerio and the other half during the school break. Lucia, as I further explain below, started this refrigerio because she noticed that waiting for the 10:30 am school break was too hard for these first-graders. They were hungry at 9 am.

Inside Lucia's classroom, a poster with the title "Plato del Bien Comer y Jarra del Buen Beber" [Eatwell Plate and Drinkwell Jug] was hung on the wall. On the plate, different foods were grouped in three sections to visually communicate the consumption levels required for a "balanced" diet. Below the plate, an image of the jug illustrated the quantities of water, milk, coffee and *refrescos* recommended for consumption. Each of these drinks appeared in different colors on the jug. Painted in blue, water occupied half of the jug with the recommendation that "6 to 8 glasses" needed to be drunk daily. The jug image conveyed the message visually: water is the healthiest drink and, therefore, we should be consumed freely.

The idea that we need to drink between six and eight glasses (around two liters) of water per day has become central to the agendas of researchers and policymakers amidst the 'fight' against obesity. The "Drinkwell Jug" represents the "beverage consumption recommendations for the Mexican population" proposed in 2008 by nutrition experts from Mexico and the United States (see Rivera et al., 2008). Framed under the energy balance discourse, these recommendations called for a decrease in energy intake from drinks as an anti-obesity measure.

Encouraging Mexicans to drink less *refrescos* and more water is a rational and much-needed piece of nutritional advice. Mexico ranks amongst the world's top consumers of *refresco*, particularly Coca-Cola (Reporte Indigo, 2017).

The implementation of NAFTA enabled the modification of packaging and advertising regulations for ultra-processed products. Changes in the legislation in land ownership and the use of water springs enabled corporations to expand their presence in Mexico. Water sales boomed, as corporations like Danone, Nestlé, Coca-Cola and PepsiCo gained the right to own and exploit water sources across Mexico in the late 1990s. In this economic environment and amidst the 'fight' against obesity, the consumption of water also became central to nutritional research. Human beings need water to function. Water comes into our bodies in different forms and from different sources. Water drank directly from a source is good, yet the idea that we need, for example, eight or more glasses of water per day has been subject to debate. In this section, I briefly discuss the science behind this nutritional recommendation in this context of the corporate dominance of water resources. It is pertinent to make clear that I am neither questioning whether water is the best hydration source nor how much water we should drink. Instead, I critically discuss how the idea that water is the healthiest hydration option has been used for the interests of corporations (for a similar sociological critique, see Hawkins, 2009; Hawkins et al., 2015; Opel, 1999; Race, 2012).

The evidence supporting the idea that we need to drink six to eight glasses of water for health purposes is limited (see Negoianu & Goldfarb, 2008; Valtin, 2002). After searching in the literature and discussing the topic with other researchers, Valtin (2002, p. R1001, original emphasis) "found no scientific reports concluding that we *all* must drink at least eight glasses of water a day".[7] For Valtin, this advice is not well supported because water does not come only from the liquid we drink from the tap or bottles. Coffee, tea, fruit and vegetables are also sources of water. Therefore, Valtin emphasizes in his conclusions that the available data suggest that "we probably are currently drinking enough and possibly more than enough" (p. R1001).

Corporate interests have directly framed both the science behind water consumption and its communication. In different ways, most research advocating for a higher and more constant consumption of water has been funded by corporations like Danone and Nestlé, the dominant players in the global bottled water business (for examples, see Armstrong & Johnson, 2018; Benelam & Wyness, 2010; Daniels & Popkin, 2010; Iglesia et al., 2015; Jéquier & Constant, 2010; Perrier et al., 2020; Piernas et al., 2014; Popkin et al., 2010; Stookey et al., 2008). Nestlé has been vocal of the message that water consumption is good for health. Its reports on water management and commercialization released in 2003 and 2007 show the centrality this message started to have for Nestlé at that time. In both reports (Nestlé, 2003, 2007), the association between water consumption and good health is emphasized, yet the use of scientific statements is more central in the 2007 report. A globally renowned nutrition researcher is featured, handling a glass of water, in a spotlight section where the scientific bases of water consumption are explained. The aim is to validate the message: "water is the most healthy option we have for the bulk of our beverage intake" (Nestlé, 2007, p. 17). The consumption of water is undoubtedly better for health than consuming artificially sweetened drinks of any kind. My intention therefore is not to question the veracity of the statement, but to spark reflection on how scientific facts can be used to advance economic interests; especially in the context of a market-driven global economy (Bakker, 2007; Ballinas & Méndez, 2006; Lemus, 2019).

The communication of water consumption science, particularly though schools, is a central element in Nestlé's water agenda. This started in 1992, when the corporation created its water division, Nestlé Water. That year, Nestlé became the sponsor of Water Education for Teachers (WET), an "international water science and education programme for classroom teachers" designed to make children aware of water and the benefits of its consumption (Nestlé, 2003). WET was designed and implemented in the U.S. and then exported to Nestlé's other key markets. Mexico was one of them. The message that water is the healthiest drink option was central to SUMA-Nutrir, the healthy lifestyles program implemented in Veracruz between the SEV and Nestlé (see Chapter 4).

At the bottom of the poster hung in the classroom at Benito Juárez Primary School, the logo of the SEV appeared in the right corner. In the left, the logo of Nestlé's Nutrir is followed by the phrase "Nestlé Niños Saludables" [Nestlé Healthy Kids]. This poster, underpinned by the 'scientific evidence' produced under Nestlé's influence and combined with other pedagogical activities described below, was one of the resources that helped replace *refrescos* with water. Another resource that helped in this task was the sugar tax. However, the decrease in consumption of *refrescos* within school time did not reflect a reduction in the total consumption of *refrescos*. What changed was the consumption patterns. The lack of infrastructure and the widespread belief that tap water is dangerous have pushed Mexican students to *buy* bottled water in schools and Coca-Cola outside.

Refrescos, the Sugar Tax and the Commodification of Water

Mexicans have a deep fondness for *refrescos*, and particularly for *Coca*, as Mexicans usually refer to Coca-Cola. In no other country around the world do people drink as much Coca as in Mexico. There is an economic and a cultural dimension for this predilection. Economically, it was enabled by the de-regulation of the market after NAFTA, which increased the flow of foreign direct investment in the country and flooded the market with energy-dense drinks made out of corn syrup, the artificial sweetener *par excellence*. The preference of Mexicans for *refrescos*—Coca in particular—over other drinks is also strong because these drinks have been widely accommodated to cultural practices (Leatherman & Goodman, 2005; Nash, 2007). Today, many Mexicans think that Coca "gives flavor to food", and therefore when eaten without drinking a Coca, food is "tasteless". The consumption of Coca has been normalized to the point that this drink is always associated with eating. Doña Martha, one of the cooks in Emiliano Zapata Primary School, evoked Coca as an indispensable component of a good meal.[8] Teachers across both schools in my fieldwork expressed, at least, a predilection for, and in other cases a deep fondness of, Coca. As the result of healthy eating policies and programs, this drink had been banned from schools. Some teachers, however, brought, or were discretely sold, bottles of Coca at the school.

Coca is omnipresent in Mexico. Wherever you go in Mexico you will be able to buy Coca, and other sugary drinks made by Coca-Cola. Market forces have enabled this to happen. Yet the high consumption of Coca-Cola products in Mexico is also the result of the communication showing why Coca-Cola is great. Advertising has had much to do with Coca-Cola becoming an important cultural signifier for people in Mexico and in increasing consumption. After the mid-1990s, the Coca-Cola logo appeared everywhere: in the red trucks delivering Coca, in tables and chairs, in parks, in TV programs, in stadiums, in schools, in myriad merchandise and in any single *tiendita* [corner store] and retail shop. It also became part of schools. Coca-Cola even created a school-based football competition called Copa Coca-Cola [Coca-Cola Cup]. Coca-Cola penetrated schools with its bottles of carbonated-sugary drinks but also through the promotion of healthy lifestyles. As I narrated in Chapter 1, the Coca-Cola sponsored programs in schools I was part of while working in Veracruz, Mexico also served as propaganda for the company.

Refrescos are not a recent element in the culture of Mexico. The industry of *refrescos* flourished in the late nineteenth/early twentieth century in diverse regions across the country (Walsh, 2018). *Refrescos* started as a luxury drink that not everyone could have, but they became gradually popularized. The consumption of these drinks therefore has been common in the last hundred years; however, consumption patterns increased drastically in the 1990s after the government loosened restrictions on packaging and pricing (Hawkes, 2002; see also Coca-Cola, 1993). I experienced the expansion of Coca-Cola while I was growing up in the 1990s. The size of *refresco* bottles became bigger and more diverse. The first bottles were made of glass and contained no more than a liter. Towards the end of the 1990s, 2 L plastic bottles had replaced the old glass bottles Coca-Cola used for its products. Today, people can buy 3 L disposable plastic bottles of Coca-Cola anywhere around Mexico. Large, red fridges with Coca-Cola logos are part of even the tiniest *tiendita* across the country.[9]

The aggressive expansion of Coca-Cola, and other drink corporations, in the last two decades (see Leatherman & Goodman, 2005; Nash, 2007) has generated an increase in the amount of *refrescos* that Mexicans drink each year (Barquera et al., 2008; Bogin et al., 2014; Nagata et al., 2011). Yet, research has linked the consumption of sugary drinks, like *refrescos*, to nutrition-related problems, such as obesity (Hu, 2013; Malik et al., 2010). In this context, increasing the availability and consumption of water has become an important component of obesity policy.

In ANSA and ENSOD it is emphasized the important role schools have in facilitating the conditions for people to replace the consumption of *refrescos* with water. In these policies, the Secretaría de Educación Pública (SEP) was urged to "equip schools" with the equipment needed to provide children with "potable and free" water. The *Lineamientos*, and programs like SUMA-Nutrir, were also aimed at encouraging the consumption of water during school time. Between 2010 and

2014, however, little was made to actively implement these policies. The implementation of the 2014 sugar tax revitalized the conversation.

The sugar tax was widely supported by researchers, members of non-government organizations and government officials. All the policymakers I interviewed in Mexico City in 2016 were actively lobbying to raise the sugar tax from 10 percent to 20 percent.[10] It could be said that they acted as part of the "pro-tax team". The bill faced fierce opposition from food and drink corporations, who came to be the "anti-tax team", in what the experienced researcher I interviewed described as a "war". In this "war" to increase the sugar tax by 10 percent, the use of evidence to demonstrate policy outcomes became crucial. The pro-tax team presented evidence to support the effectiveness of the sugar tax. The other band presented evidence to challenge this point. The industry-supported evidence nonetheless was produced under a clear conflict of interest.

NGOs actively lobbying for actions against obesity proposed earmarking the revenue raised from the sugar tax to fund fountains in schools; an argument that became a flagship cause to justify the public health outcomes the tax would have. However, as they told me, this was not a popular proposal for the government.

Between 2015 and 2018, the federal government assigned this funding for water fountains in schools. Each education authority in the states received the funding through a program called Bebederos Escolares [Water Fountains in Schools], managed by the department of infrastructure within the organization. However, the number of schools that received the benefits of this program was limited. Many schools, Emiliano Zapata and Benito Juárez primary schools included, did not even know this program existed.

The activists I interviewed also had interesting views on the relationship between the access to water and private interests. Adolfo, the director of Anti-obesity Action, was a fervent defendant of the sugar tax and of water fountains in schools. At the same time, he also considered that the problem of water availability could be solved by relying on corporate resources. "If Coca-Cola and Pepsi have the largest distribution and commercialization networks in Mexico", Adolfo said, "which make their products available in places where there are not even hospitals or other services, then, these networks should be used to increase the availability of water". Although he expressed deep concerns about corporate involvement in obesity policymaking, Adolfo did not seem unsatisfied with corporations supplying the bottled water that most Mexicans are forced to buy because of the state not providing clean tap water. "If you have potable water as part of your product portfolio, then sell potable water as well", he concluded. As Adolfo suggested, and as can be corroborated in multiple sales reports (Euromonitor International, 2018a, 2018b; statista, 2013, n.d.), drinks corporations have expanded their "product portfolio" significantly. Water has become a particularly crucial commodity in their portfolios. And given the lack of infrastructure in Mexico, corporations have become the providers of drinkable water for the entire population, which has translated into making profit.

The members of Anti-Obesity Coalition I interviewed, Ernesto and Nadia, were more aware of the commodification process that has accompanied attempts to increase the availability and consumption of water. Ernesto considered that access to "potable and quality water" should be more balanced across the market. Unlike Adolfo, who sometimes assumed that water needed to be bought in bottles, Ernesto showed some degree of reflection about the inappropriateness of buying water in bottles. "If you have to buy a bottle of water, which is not the ideal", he said, "the price of water should be lower than the price of *refrescos*". Nadia made a more critical point that challenged Adolfo's view about the corporate provision of bottled water. From her perspective, the fact that Coca-Cola had started to "produce water" as well as *refrescos* was good from a public health point of view. However, Nadia considered that this shift from one drink to another "is strategically aimed to make greater profits". As global reports on bottled water sales and the data that I discuss below reveal, Nadia was right.

Water and Corporate Profits: A View from Schools

Schools have been tasked with the responsibility of promoting the consumption of water and making it available for students. Under the material conditions described so far, this is a complex task. When people in my fieldwork talked about water consumption in schools, they always assumed that one needed to buy bottled water. To a great extent, they perceived tap water as "dangerous" and corporations to be the obvious distributors of bottled water. These ideas are so rooted among most Mexicans that none of my interviewees problematized why they should be dependent on, and pay money to, corporations to obtain water. In fact, most of them looked favourably on the fact that Coca-Cola was selling water instead of *refrescos* in schools.

An emblematic example of this situation was provided by Alicia, the secretary of education in Veracruz, during our interview in late June 2016. By the time I interviewed her, Alicia had worked in different positions within the SEV for more than 40 years. She had started her career as a primary school teacher in the late 1960s and climbed up the ladder of the educational bureaucracy in the state. There was not a single position within the SEV—from classroom teacher to superintendent, to department director—that Alicia had not done. This gave Alicia a deep inside-knowledge of the workings and politics of education, food sales included, in the state.

Alicia described at length the difficulties in disseminating the *Lineamientos* and in making schools to comply with this policy. She also highlighted the "important" partnerships the SEV had stablished with "food enterprises", which contributed to enabling children to access healthier food and drink options in schools. For example, in recent years FEMSA, Coca-Cola's largest bottler and distributor in Latin America, has agreed, Alicia explained to me, to "introduce water, water instead of *refrescos*". The commitment of this corporation was such, Alicia stated vehemently, that they were "not simply introducing teas, or all those [sugary] products that are more of the same; no, they are introducing water".

In Chapter 4, I demonstrated how corporate-funded programs promoting healthy lifestyles in schools have worked to expand a corporate perspective about health, nutrition and self-care. These same programs have also contributed in encouraging Mexicans to buy, at least in school hours, fewer *refrescos* and more bottled water. Alicia considered this a "success". Undoubtedly, it is an important achievement. However, in Alicia's words it is implicit the extent to which paying for water has been normalized. Interested by Alicia's optimistic perspective on public–corporate partnerships, I asked her whether she perceived any potential negative consequences. With a sly smile and a stentorian voice, she said:

> Well, Nestlé, for example, has allowed us to develop a program that has had an incredible impact in the schools. But what can I say about the complaints from the pseudo-intellectuals who say, 'How is that possible?' Let's see, let's see, let's see... We don't have to sell any product from that corporation in the schools. You can visit the schools and you will not see a single product from Nestlé. They ask *nothing from us* [her emphasis]. They only offer us a program that we review, that is adequate and that helps us. FEMSA is our sponsor in a program called Coordenadas para Vivir [Coordinates for Living]. They [FEMSA] have never told us... instead, we use that approach to ask them not to sell some products. Coca-Cola is not sold in any school in Veracruz. You will not find Coca-Cola in *any school* [her emphasis]. You can come here and put it here (points the desk) if you find Coca-Cola in one school. They don't sell that; *they just sell water* [my emphasis] ...

Alicia was right. Neither Coca nor any other *refrescos* were available in the schools that I visited during my fieldwork.[11] However, Coca-Cola, the corporation, was present in schools, but now with different products like water and, to a lesser extent, juices. The fact that Mexicans have to buy the water they drink is so obvious that Alicia did not perceive any problem in having Coca-Cola and other corporations promote water consumption. She did not perceive any issue in having these corporations sell bottled water either. What mattered was that water was available for purchase in schools. At Benito Juárez Primary School, for example, Ciel garrafones, 600 mL bottles of Ciel water and Frutsis[12] were delivered to Nutrilandia twice a week. In most classrooms, there was usually a 20 L garrafón of Ciel water that was usually bought out of the students' daily contribution.

At Emiliano Zapata Primary School, Coca-Cola's presence was not as strong. Only a couple of cases of 600 mL Ciel bottles were delivered each week. The school community tried to be less dependent on Coca-Cola's resources and to ameliorate the negative effects implicit in the commodification of water. Water used to cook and to prepare *aguas frescas* [fresh fruit water] in the kitchen was sourced from a local bottling company called Xallapan. Inside some classrooms, there were also some Xallapan garrafones upside-down in dispensers that kept the water cool. The cost of Xallapan garrafones was considerably cheaper than Coca-Cola's brand, Ciel. Also, the school community sought ways to make bottles of water available at the lowest price.

For instance, on a hot morning in June 2016, I observed the principal Andrés arrive in his office with seven cases of bottles of water. He cut the pallet's stretch wrap and placed the bottles in the fridge. Previously, the principal had told me that Ciel water, delivered to the school, was too expensive, so he had considered buying bottled water from U.S. wholesale retailers like Costco or Sam's Club. The bottled water that day had been bought from Costco, and although Andrés had driven 40 km to Veracruz City, the trip was worth it. Andrés wanted to lower the price per bottle from 6 to 5 pesos because students were buying water constantly due to the extreme heat. However, this decision had a negative impact on the school's provision of food. The small income from bottled water sales was usually used to cover the revenue deficit from the kitchen (see Chapters 1 and 5).

In one of my last visits to Emiliano Zapata Primary School, I interviewed Andrés in his office. Having heard various opinions about the need to increase water consumption in schools as a public health measure, my penultimate question touched on this point. In particular, I asked the principal about the water fountain program released at the same time as the sugar tax. I wanted to know if the principal was aware of the program and whether he perceived there to be a benefit in having a water fountain in the school. He answered:

> Children already consume water, and they consume it to a great extent, actually. The evidence is that I sell water here in the office, which I try to make the best quality water at the cheapest price. If we had the filters, if we had the water fountains each classroom wouldn't need to get their garrafón. I would not need to sell water here either. Water would become cheap. Children would not have to pay for water anymore. It would be a great help for the parents.

Sadly, the program to provide schools with water fountains using funds from the sugar tax did not benefit many Mexican schools. As is usual in the Mexican context, the government allocated funds to the program, but the fountains to provide clean, free water for students were rarely installed. In a manifestation of corruption, the money never reached its final destination. According to the Mexican Audit Office (Auditoría Superior de la Federación, 2018, p. 9), by 2018, only 37.1 percent of the promised water fountains had been installed in schools since 2015. In the 2016–2017 school year, for example, the government assigned "1,113,572.9 billion pesos to pay for the installation and maintenance of 8,000 water fountains". However, by the end of that year none of those water fountains had been installed. The idea that taxing sugar would directly translate into greater use of tap water in Mexican schools, and, therefore, into a public health achievement, was great on paper. But for the school community, this promise did not become true. Meanwhile, students have to keep buying Coca-Cola, PepsiCo or Nestlé bottled water in schools.

Decreasing the consumption of sugary drinks among the Mexican population is an important strategy. Few countries in the world drink *refrescos* as much as people in Mexico. However, the good intentions of this aim of anti-obesity policy fall apart when, for the historical and political reasons explained above, the "producers" and "distributors" of bottled water are profiting in the name of making people 'healthy'. The *dispositif of healthy lifestyles*, I suggest, has connected the discourse of water as the 'healthiest' drink with corporate profits. This link has been made possible due to the discourse's materialization into practice. How have corporations used the promotion of healthy lifestyles to facilitate the commodification of water in Mexico? This question can be understood and answered by looking at day-to-day health-promotion work in schools.

Teaching Bottled Water Consumption

On one of my last days of fieldwork, I was sitting in the dining area during the break at Emiliano Zapata Primary School. A slim, well-groomed student sat next to me and opened his lunchbox. He was one of the few children who did not usually eat food from the kitchen. Every morning at break time, his mum delivered a lunchbox and some money. "I have 15 pesos. I'm going to buy fruit and use 6 pesos to buy a juice... or maybe water, because I have physical education", the boy said. I asked him why he did not bring water from home instead of buying a bottle there. "Because I always lose the [reusable] bottles, so it's easier for my parents to just give me money to buy a drink from the school", he replied. This student, like Carlos, the child with the whole-grain sandwich, differentiated between the health properties of drinking water and consuming sugary drinks. Carlos also knew where the right place was to consume each drink. At school, he only drank water from his bottle, but given that he "loved sugar", Carlos had *refrescos* daily at home.

The regulation of what drinks are allowed to be commercialized in schools has undoubtedly been successful in making Mexican students drink more bottled water. However, banning, or trying to ban, *refrescos* from schools has not been the only reason why the consumption of bottled water has increased among students. A key driver in the water-consumption equation has been teachers' health-promotion work, motivated by the national curriculum, policies like the *Lineamientos* and programs like SUMA-Nutrir. In this section, I show how the *dispositif of healthy lifestyles* has shaped pedagogical practices in schools that have materialized in an increased consumption of bottled water in Mexico. Particularly, I show how Mexican students have been taught that drinking water is 'healthy' and that, consequently, they should constantly consume it. I build my case drawing on observations and interviews at Benito Juárez Primary School, where I observed the association, described in Euromonitor International's (2018a) report on soft drinks, between the "interesting growth" in bottled water sales and the "constant reminder" to Mexicans that drinking water is one of the most recommended 'healthy' habits.

In ENSOD (p. 85), the need for "[p]romoting the availability and consumption of plain potable water in schools" was highlighted as the responsibility of federal and state-level education authorities. The *Lineamientos 2014* (p. 3), on its part, emphasized that schools should promote "the importance of consuming plain potable water as the first hydration option". Therefore, schools regulated, as I described above, what could be sold and drunk during school time, but also adopted other strategies to make children drink more water. At Benito Juárez Primary School, for instance, the "Drinkwell Jug" was painted on the white wall in front of Nutrilandia (see Figure 1.2 in Chapter 1) and posters were displayed inside classrooms. These material objects that communicated the message of water as the 'healthiest' drink option were also complemented by the decisive work of teachers who promoted water consumption as part of their everyday teaching practices. The range of activities that Lucia implemented to take care of her students' health help me show this point.

The refrigerio, the 10-minute refreshment break at 9 am that Lucia implemented in her First-Year classroom, is an example of how teachers aided to change the consumption of *refrescos* for water within school hours. Lucia started the refrigerio in 2009 as a classroom policy to address two issues. The first, and more important for her, was that not all students came to school having had breakfast at home. "Some students have at least a smoothie, others have coffee but", she said, "there are other students who come without any food in their stomachs, they just wake up and come to school; so, they are hungry". The lack of food before school impacts negatively on students. "When we are hungry", as Lucia stated, "we're just thinking about food, about satisfying that need", which affects students' ability to focus, engage and learn in the classroom.[13] Lucia was conscious that the refrigerio at 9 am was not "a formal breakfast", but at least she was doing what was in their hands to care for the students. Lucia was the only teacher implementing a refrigerio at Benito Juárez Primary School. No one had asked her to do it, and there was no policy document, corporate program or curriculum material that asked teachers to implement this kind of strategy. However, as teachers usually do, Lucia took this step because she had perceived the need among her students.

The second reason for Lucia to start with the refrigerio was to address the excessive consumption of ultra-processed products by students:

> One day, a kid brought Coca in his [reusable] bottle. I mean, I don't think there's anything wrong with that drink, but I do consider that Coca is a drink for adults and it's not good for breakfast. So, when I noticed that the kid had brought Coca in his bottle; so I opened the bottled, smelled it, and proved that the bottle had been filled up with Coca. That was when I said, '*Yes*', I said, 'Well, I have to implement the refrigerio, I have to talk to the parents, because the culture, the habits are not the right ones'.

While Lucia did not follow any directions in developing the refrigerio, she used this strategy to teach curriculum content about the importance of drinking water and eating 'healthily'. This more regulatory-oriented aim of the refrigerio gained relevance in the context of the deployment of the *Lineamientos 2010* between 2011 and 2013. Simultaneously, this strategy came to be paired with SUMA-Nutrir during the two years the program was underway in the school.

The refrigerio worked as a powerful pedagogical device that Lucia developed to take care of her students' wellbeing, and to teach nutrition and health content.

However, during the two years of the SUMA-Nutrir roll-out and its close monitoring in the school, the refrigerio became a tool to promote healthy lifestyles. In those two years, Lucia tried to connect SUMA-Nutrir's content with what she was teaching about health promotion. She also worked in-depth on promoting the intake of plain water. "I created a daily record, a nutrition record to register what students brought daily". While Lucia did not explicitly mention it, the refrigerio and her other health-promotion activities became a kind of surveillance tool (in the sense that I problematized in Chapter4) after SUMA-Nutrir arrived at the school. Lucia's response to my question about whether she had implemented the refrigerio with other grades provides an example:

> I always implement the refrigerio strategy with the little kids, I mean with first- and second-grade students. With older students, from third to sixth grades, I don't do it. What I do, older kids are already used to waiting to eat until 10:30 am, when the school break starts, so I just try to encourage them to have breakfast at home, to bring good food for the break and to drink plain water. What I do is, we have daily challenges. We collect statistics about the days when students bring water. We usually start the school year with [students bringing] juices, Frutsis and other things like that, and usually by the end of the year the kids get use to bringing water, plain water. We try to gradually make them change the habit of consuming so much sugar, at least at school.

Lucia was really invested in making her students consume fewer sugary drinks and more plain water. From what I observed in the classroom and from what I knew about her, Lucia was a very professional, committed and well-resourced teacher. I have no doubts that her desire to create 'healthier' habits in the students was legitimate. Indeed, Lucia considered education to be holistic in its approach and that it should teach students to collaboratively take care of their health. "I think that teachers' work is not only about teaching children to read, for example. It is about trying to offer a comprehensive education for the kids", she responded passionately, when I asked why she was so engaged in procuring her students' health. However, at least in regard to teaching children that water is healthier than *refrescos*, Lucia never problematized why water should be bought and consumed from bottles, instead of simply drunk from the tap.

The historical belief held by Mexicans that tap water is "dangerous" undoubtedly plays a role here. Mexicans have been taught for many years to avoid running water and instead to opt for bottled, or boiled, water. Therefore, it should not come as a surprise that Lucia, like all the teachers who I spoke with, did not envisage that any other form of water consumption was possible. In this context, it could be said that the very well-intentioned actions Lucia developed to make water more available for students, and to teach them the importance of preferring water over *refrescos*, were successful from a pedagogical point of view, but they also helped to increase the profits of corporations. Saying this does not mean that I consider teachers to be passive actors who are just following directions or overwhelmed by an unchallenged power structure. Instead, teachers do more than teaching water consumption. They also design and implement small, but significant, strategies on the ground to give students access to water, despite the lack of state support.

Furthermore, making students avoid the consumption of carbonated-sugary drinks *inside* the school was not an easy task for teachers. The *Lineamientos 2010* helped substantially, banning the sale of *refrescos* from school, which is undoubtedly one of its most important merits. However, this policy did not impede students from bringing Coca from *outside* and thereby increasing the influx of this drink through reusable bottles. Both the curriculum and SUMA-Nutrir aided in providing valuable information about the negative effects of *refrescos* and the health benefits of drinking water. As I discussed in this section, elements from all these strategies were brought together by Lucia, who turned the refrigerio into a surveillance mechanism to gradually convince her students of not drinking *refrescos* in the school. As Carlos' story shows, she was partially successful. Nevertheless, all the efforts of this teacher were unfruitful in undoing Carlos's fascination for Coca, the drink that this little seven-year-old had as many times as he could throughout the day outside of the school. In the end, he, like millions of Mexicans, is dependent on Coca-Cola to satiate his thirst, either from water or from Coca.

Bottled Water: The Elephant in the Room?

Increasing the availability and consumption of water has been one of the most noticeable outcomes of healthy lifestyles. The discourses around water consumption that frame obesity policy, like the ones making up the "Drinkwell Jug", were dispersed through programs and became tangible practices in schools. Emiliano Zapata and Benito Juárez primary schools swapped the sale of *refrescos* for bottled water, driven by the *Lineamientos* and the messages of SUMA-Nutrir. However, the water stories from within the day-to-day lives of these schools showcase the complex politics behind the desire to make Mexicans drink more water in the name of 'health'. Teachers, education authorities and principals have struggled to increase the availability of water in schools. Having Coca-Cola's fridges full of bottles of water instead of Coca proved that schools were willing and able to offer healthier drinking options to the students. Nonetheless, that fridge also shows how corporations, both producers and retailers, have benefited extensively from the idea that water is the 'healthiest' drink and, therefore, needs to be consumed regularly.

The consumption of Coca is so deeply rooted in Mexican culture that efforts to change children's taste for it has been only partially successful. What has changed are consumption patterns. As Carlos' comments show, water has become the drink at school, but Coca is still the preferred option at home. Banning *refrescos* from schools has, partially, decreased their consumption *inside* those spaces, and health-promotion work has made children aware that *refrescos* are bad for their health. Nonetheless, neither restrictions nor interventions have modified children's affection for Coca.

This point was clearly made by a fourth-grade student at Benito Juárez Primary School, when we were chatting on the school's patio during recess. The student told me what he regularly bought from Nutrilandia with the money he was given. "Sometimes, when I have 30 pesos, I buy a *quesadilla*, a bottle of water and a *cochinada* [shitty food]".[14] As our conversation progressed, the boy said he usually drank a lot of Coca. "Which is healthier?", I asked, comparing water and Coca. "Water!", he shouted. I immediately asked what he liked more. "Coca. I have around four glasses of Coca a day. I especially like Coca for breakfast", he said. Before he ran away, this kid said he loved to have Coca while eating, because "water makes food tasteless".

As a Mexican myself, I have endlessly heard—from family, friends, colleagues and strangers—the claim that food *without* Coca is *tasteless*. Most of the people in this research shared this perspective. For this reason, teachers used to say humorously that the ban on Coca in schools did not apply to them. Coca was always available for them. I am raising this point not intending to be judgmental of teachers, but to emphasize the extent to which Coca has become a sort of (unfortunate?) culinary necessity for Mexicans. Of course, as I have discussed previously, this change in taste and diet has been facilitated by market-driven reforms and aggressive marketing.

The change in the consumption of Coca for water is good. However, it is problematic when both products are sold by the same corporation. *Refrescos* and bottled water are, for example, a win–win enterprise for Coca-Cola. It comes as no surprise that this corporation has been deeply invested in promoting water consumption through the use of its brand. During my school visit with Victoria in late May 2016 (Chapter 4), I saw a water fountain at the other end of the patio as we were exiting the school. When Victoria stopped to talk with a group of mothers about the need to avoid selling *tamales* for breakfast, I decided to have a closer look at this rare artefact within Mexican schools. Predictably, the water fountain was not working. What amazed me, however, was the logo of the Fundación Coca-Cola [Coca-Cola Foundation] that I discovered on the fountain's top-right corner.

Initially, I did not pay much attention to that event. I interpreted that useless water fountain as just another example of another project for schools that had been launched and later abandoned. However, as I made more sense of the connections between healthy lifestyles, water, corporations and neoliberalism in Mexico, I was able to understand the deep symbolism of that water fountain. It was not useless, at least not for Coca-Cola. Quite the opposite: the fountain epitomizes—and I am deliberately using the present tense here—the extent to which the myriad discourses and practices triggered by the 'fight' against obesity have allowed the expansion of corporate interests among the Mexican population. Emblematically, the fountain portrays *the* spring of power which is the source of the knowledges about the obesity problem and its solutions.

The profitable bottled water market for Coca-Cola, PepsiCo, Nestlé and Danone has not appeared magically. The wave of neoliberal policies implemented in the late 1980s contributed to increasing the profitability of bottled water in

Mexico. As an example, these policies materialized years later, in the *Ley de Aguas Nacionales* 1992 [*National Water Law* 1992] promulgated under the Salinas administration. This law enabled the rise of the bottled water industry by allowing a transfer of water rights from the public to the private sphere (Nash, 2007; Wilder, 2010). In this respect, Nash (2007, pp. 632–633) argues that during the presidency of Vicente Fox, who was the former director of Coca-Cola in Mexico, the "drive to privatize rights to exploit groundwater and make it available to foreign companies surged", granting "the right to exploit more groundwater in a country than ever before". The Mexican government has not only relinquished its obligation to make tap water available for human consumption, it has also laid the groundwork for corporations to profit from the increasing consumption of bottled water, as motivated by healthy lifestyles.

Scholars have argued that the adoption of neoliberalism as a mode of government has facilitated the commodification of water at a global scale (Bakker, 2007; Swyngedouw, 2005). Others, including activists, have argued that, given the vitality of water for almost all human activities, from hydration to the production of commodities like bottled water, and the scarcity of the resource, a "war" to own and control water resources has started globally (Lemus, 2019; Shiva, 2016). In Mexico, for example, a social conflict has arisen in Santa Rita Tlahuapan, a community in central Mexico, after Nestlé was granted control over local springs. From this water source, Nestlé sources one-third of the water required to prepare many of its products. Sta. María, Nestlé's water brand, is bottled in this community, which has had a negative impact on the population's already-limited access to water (Lemus, 2019).

Teachers, students, parents and cooks in Mexican schools have been caught amidst this complex, politically and economically motivated management of water. They have been pushed to look for options to ensure the availability and consumption of water in school time. The way in which water was made available at Emiliano Zapata and Benito Juárez primary schools resonated with Adolfo's proposal of relying on corporations' distribution networks. The success of this strategy has been to simply change the consumption of one product for another sold by the same corporation. Thus, drinking water for 'health' purposes becomes an economic imperative. Of course, I support children having the option of buying water rather than *refrescos* at school, but it would be preferable if political efforts were made to facilitate access to free, clean water, as is stipulated in Mexican and international laws. Otherwise, water becomes merchandise that increases the profits of corporations and strengthens their presence in schools under the idea of healthy lifestyles. Perhaps it is unsurprising that water has just began trading on Wall Street, just like other commodities such as gold or oil (Chipman, 2020).

The existence, and the nature, of the two *Lineamientos*, ANSA, ENSOD and the corporate–public programs that I have described in this research could be explained in the context of the economic liberalization and political transformations that Mexico has experienced since the 1980s. Therefore, as I elaborated earlier following Foucault (2007), I have come to consider ANSA, ENSOD and the two *Lineamientos* as a form to "safeguard" the Mexican population from the voracious negative effects introduced by the neoliberal form of government. The packaging and marketing regulations for ultra-processed foods and drinks that were loosened in the early 1990s facilitated the expansion of Coca-Cola, Nestlé, Walmart, PepsiCo and other corporations. Therefore, the "health technocrats", based on a public health approach that positions health as part of the market, developed actions to shift the blame from structural changes onto individual failures. This has been the preferred approach to ameliorate the health problems that, as a large body of research has shown, were introduced by neoliberalism in Mexico.

It would be erroneous to claim that anti-obesity policies and programs have been useless. They have had diverse consequences for different actors, as I have shown in this book. If we take water consumption as an example, it could be argued that the discourses and practices of the *dispositif of healthy lifestyles* have successfully stopped the intake of *refrescos* and increased the amount of water that students consume in schools. However, while they have pushed students to *buy* water at schools in the name of healthy lifestyles, anti-obesity policies and programs have been unable to change the affection that children, and most of the Mexican population, have for Coca. Therefore, increasing the consumption of water inside schools has been a win–win situation for Coca-Cola, and has equally generated vast profit for other food and drink corporations.

Water has allowed me to connect discourses, discursive arrangements and material practices to show how corporations have used the water–'healthy lifestyles' connection to push their agendas. Cutting calories from drinks has been deemed a successful anti-obesity action. In an ideal world, having Mexican children drinking less Coca in schools would be a reason to celebrate. However, that optimism breaks down when we see that, enabled by the *dispositif of healthy lifestyles*, Coca-Cola and other corporations have diversified their revenue sources. Thus, in the name of making a 'healthy' population, they have also profited vastly from selling millions of bottles of water to a thirsty population.[15]

Conclusion

The growth in bottled water consumption in Mexico has been a success for the obesity policy agenda. ANSA, ENSOD, the *Lineamientos 2010* and the *Lineamientos 2014* task schools with encouraging people to avoid sugary drinks, mainly *refrescos*, and to increase the consumption of water, deemed the best hydration option. SUMA-Nutrir translated this policy mandate into practice through several health-promotion activities in schools. Under these frameworks, teachers at Emiliano Zapata and Benito Juárez primary schools actively promoted water consumption among students. Combined, these actions have pushed Mexicans to buy more water. While I acknowledge that water is healthier than *refrescos*, the fact that Mexicans are buying more bottled water does not necessarily mean that they are 'healthier'. Instead, in a country that for many years has lacked the infrastructure and the political will to provision its population with clean, safe tap water, the high consumption of bottled water has to be understood as a success for corporations rather than a public health triumph for the Mexican people.

Notes

1 In English, a sandwich can be made from multiple types of breads and be filled with a wide range of fresh, cooked and pickled ingredients. In Mexico this logic does not apply. A "sandwich" in Mexico will always be made of white, off-the-shelf bread, filled with (industrial) ham and yellow cheese. In the story, Carlos is distinguishing his consumption with the emphasis on the sandwich being "whole-grain", instead of white-only bread. The largest producer and seller of industrial bread in Mexico, BIMBO, advertises its wholegrain-range breads as 'healthier'.

2 As I elaborate throughout this book, Mexican people are avid consumers of *refrescos*, particularly of Coca-Cola. The consumption of carbonated-sugary drinks has substantially increased in the Global South from the early 2000s (Barquera et al., 2008; Russell et al., 2022; Stuckler et al., 2012).

3 I consulted the report's executive summary online in late 2018. The report was updated in March 2019 and then in 2020. The link for this report that I have added in my list of references updates automatically. Therefore, if the reader accesses the provided link, they will be directed to the 2020, or possibly 2021, version of the report. I did not purchase the full 2018 Soft Drinks in Mexico report because its price was around 2,000 USD.

4 Research has demonstrated a link between the tax implementation and a slight decrease in the purchase of these drinks between 2014 and 2016 (Colchero et al., 2017). Other analyses have situated this decrease as the result of multiple interconnected factors (Álvarez-Sánchez, 2018). For example, the sugar tax also applied to sweetened, packaged snack foods, which also impacted the day-to-day spending of the population, making it more expensive to consume both sugary drinks and packaged snacks. All the studies on the effectiveness of the sugar tax have focused on *refrescos*, ruling out how the consumption of industrialized juices, teas, sport and energy drinks and flavored milks has moved along with the tax. Platforms reporting on sales provide an estimate of how the increase in sugary drinks other than *refrescos* and bottled water have gone up as the sale of the latter is going down. The reports mention both the tax on sugar and the promotion of healthy lifestyles as important drivers in this change and recommend corporations to further innovate and expand their portfolio of products.

5 Multiple studies have shown that tap water in Mexico does not usually meet the criteria to be safe for human consumption. For an example, see Mazari-Hiriart et al. (2010).

6 The source is in Spanish. The translation is mine.

7 Valtin (2002, p. R1001, original emphasis) clarifies that his findings apply to "*healthy* adults in a *temperate* climate, performing, at most, *mild* exercise".

8 In her research on women's work, intra-household dynamics and food habits in three communities in Mozambique, Stevano (2014, pp. 245–247) describes how people in these communities see *refrescos* (this same term is used in Mozambique to refer to carbonated-sugary drinks) as a "good source" of vitamins and to therefore be "good for children's health". This representation of these products, Stevano suggests, is the result of aggressive marketing and the class distinction that comes with their consumption.

9 The annual reports from Coca-Cola offers good evidence of its market expansion and the gradual conquest of the *tienditas*. Pictures across these reports show, for instance, how small stores started to be painted in all over with Coca-Cola logos and colors. The Coca-Cola (1993) annual report offers a good example.

10 For the broad, anthropologically-influenced definition of policymaker I have adopted in this research, see footnote 17 in Chapter 1.

11 I only visited five schools during my fieldwork. I cannot say that the same happens in all Veracruz schools. However, from my own experience within the SEV, I consider that Coca is not usually available for sale in the cooperativas escolares. However, other drinks from Coca-Cola and other corporations are widely available.
12 Frutsi is a brand of juices for children owned by Coca-Cola in Mexico. Frutsis are a very popular and widely available drink in Mexican primary schools.
13 For a meta-analysis of the relationship between breakfast consumption and school performance among children, see Rampersaud et al. (2005).
14 This is a difficult word to translate. The student is making reference to chips, candies and other ultra-processed foods.
15 Producing bottled water is cheaper than producing *refrescos* (Gleick, 2005), so the higher consumption of bottled water has translated into greater profits for corporations. In this regard, Gleick (2005, p. 23) argues that even after the "cost of labor, bottling, plastic bottles, transportation and marketing", bottled water "remains a product with high profits", which has encouraged corporations to push bottled water production and sales.

References

Aboites-Aguilar, L. (2004). De bastión a amenaza. Agua, políticas públicas y cambio institucional en México, 1947–2001 [From bastion to threat. Water, public policies and institutional change in Mexico 1947–2001]. In B. Graizbord & J. Arroyo-Alengadre (eds.), *El futuro del agua en México* [*The future of water in Mexico*] (pp. 89–113). COLMEX/UdG/UCLA PROFMEX.

Aboites-Aguilar, L., Birricha-Gardida, D., & Garay-Trejo, J. A. (2010). El manejo de las aguas Mexicanas en el Siglo XX [Water management in 20th century Mexico]. In B. Jiménez-Cisneros, M. L. Torrgrosa y Amerntia, & L. Aboites-Aguilar (eds.), *El agua en México: Cauces y encauces* [*Water in Mexico: Riverbeds and directions*] (pp. 21–49). Academia Mexicana de Ciencias.

Acuerdo Nacional para la Salud Alimentaria. Estrategia contra el sobrepeso y la obesidad [*National Agreement for Nutritional Health. Strategy against overweight and obesity*] (ANSA) (2010). Secretaría de Salud, México.

Álvarez -Sánchez, C. (2018). *Mexicans' consumption of taxed sugar-sweetened beverages and the psychosocial determinants of consumption in the context of the 2014 Sugar-Sweetened Beverage Tax—a mixed methods study* [Doctor of Philosophy, Columbia University, New York].

Armstrong, L. E., & Johnson, E. C. (2018). Water intake, water balance, and the elusive daily water requirement. *Nutrients*, 10(12), 1928. https://doi.org/10.3390/nu10121928.

Auditoría Superior de la Federación (2018). *Auditoría de cumplimiento financiero: 2017–1-11MDE-15-0174-2018 174-DS* [*Financial audit of: 2017–1-11MDE-15-0174-2018 174-DS*]. https://www.asf.gob.mx/Trans/Informes/IR2017a/Documentos/Auditorias/2017_0174_a.pdf.

Bakker, K. (2007). The "commons" versus the "commodity": Alter-globalization, anti-privatization and the human right to water in the Global South. *Antipode*, 39(3), 430–455. https://doi.org/10.1111j.1467-8330.2007.00534.x.

Ballinas, V., & Méndez, E. (2006). Fox triplicó las concesiones del líquido; Coca-Cola y Nestlé, las beneficiadas: PRD [Fox tripled water concessions to benefit Coca-Cola and Nestlé: PRD]. *La Jornada*. https://www.jornada.com.mx/2006/03/17/index.php?section=sociedad&article=050n1soc.

Barquera, S., Hernandez-Barrera, L., Tolentino, M. L., Espinosa, J., Ng, S. W., Rivera, J. A., & Popkin, B. M. (2008). Energy intake from beverages is increasing among Mexican

adolescents and adults. *The Journal of Nutrition*, 138(12), 2454–2461. https://doi.
org/10.3945/jn.108.092163.

Barragán, D. (2015). El agua embotellada: Un despojo que inició hace 30 años [Bottled
water: An assault that started 30 years ago]. SinEmbargo. https://www.sinembargo.
mx/24-04-2015/1316594.

Benelam, B., & Wyness, L. (2010). Hydration and health: A review. *Nutrition Bulletin*, 35
(1), 3–25. https://doi.org/10.1111/j.1467-3010.2009.01795.x.

Bogin, B., Azcorra, H., Wilson, H. J., Vázquez-Vázquez, A., Avila-Escalante, M. L., Cas-
tillo-Burguete, M. T., Varela-Silva, I., & Dickinson, F. (2014). Globalization and children's diets: The case of Maya of Mexico and Central America. *Anthropological Review*,
77(1), 11–32. https://doi.org/10.2478/anre-2014-0002.

Chipman, K. (2020). California water futures begin trading amid fear of scarcity. *Bloomberg
Green*. https://www.bloomberg.com/news/articles/2020-12-06/water-futures-to-start-
trading-amid-growing-fears-of-scarcity.

Coca-Cola (1993). *The Coca-Cola Company 1993 Annual Report*. Available from the
author on request.

Colchero, M. A., Rivera-Dommarco, J., Popkin, B. M., & Ng, S. W. (2017). In Mexico,
evidence of sustained consumer response two years after implementing a Sugar-Sweetened Beverage Tax. *Health Affairs*, 36(3), 564–571. https://doi.org/10.1377/hlthaff.
2016.1231.

Daniels, M. C., & Popkin, B. M. (2010). Impact of water intake on energy intake and
weight status: A systematic review. *Nutrition Revews*, 68(9), 505–521. https://doi.org/
10.1111/j.1753-4887.2010.00311.x.

Delgado-Ramos, G. C., Meza-Velarde, A., Chávez-Mejía, A., Navarro-González, I., &
Ávila-Calero, S. (2014). Estudio de país: Una revisión de casos [A study of the Mexican
case]. In G. C. Delgado-Ramos (ed.), *Apropiación de agua, medio ambiente y obesidad:
Los impactos del negocio de bebidas embotelladas en México* [*Water appropriation, the
environment and obesity: The impact of bottled drinks in Mexico*] (pp. 75–165). Universidad Nacional Autónoma de México.

Estrada-Vivas, L. Y. (2016). *Los rostros del agua embotellada en México: Por qué somos los
mayores bebedores de este problema?* [*The faces of bottled water: Why are Mexicans the
global largest consumers of this problem?*]Centro de Investigación y Docencia Económicas, A.C. Ciudad de México.

*Estrategia Nacional para la Prevención y el Control del Sobrepeso, la Obesidad y la Diabetes
[National Strategy for the Prevention and Control of Overweight, Obesity and Diabetes]
(ENSOD)* (2013). Secretaría de Salud, México.

Euromonitor International (2018a). *Country report: Bottled water in Mexico*. Retrieved 28
February from https://www.euromonitor.com/bottled-water-in-mexico/report.

Euromonitor International (2018b). Soft drinks in Mexico. Executive summary. https://
www.euromonitor.com/soft-drinks-in-mexico/report.

Gleick, P. H. (2005). The myth and reality of bottled water. In P. H. Gleick (ed.), *The
World's Water 2004–2005: The biennial report on freshwater resources, part 8* (pp. 17–44).
Island Press.

Greene, J. (2018). Bottled water in Mexico: The rise of a new access to water paradigm. *Wiley
Interdisciplinary Reviews: Water*, 5(4), e1286. https://doi.org/10.1002/wat2.1286.

Hawkes, C. (2002). Marketing activities of global soft drink and fast food companies in
emerging markets: A review. In *Globalization, diets and noncommunicable diseases*.
World Health Organization. https://apps.who.int/iris/bitstream/handle/10665/
42609/9241590416.pdf;sequence=1.

Hawkins, G. (2009). The politics of bottled water: Assembling bottled water as brand, waste and oil. *Journal of Cultural Economy*, 2(1–2),183–195. https://doi.org/10.1080/17530350903064196.

Hawkins, G., Potter, E., & Race, K. (2015). *Plastic water: The social and material life of bottled water*. The MIT Press.

Hu, F. B. (2013). Resolved: There is sufficient scientific evidence that decreasing sugar-sweetened beverage consumption will reduce the prevalence of obesity and obesity-related diseases. *Obesity Reviews*, 14(8), 606–619. https://doi.org/10.1111/obr.12040.

Iglesia, I., Guelinckx, I., De Miguel-Etayo, P. M., González-Gil, E. M., Salas-Salvadó, J., Kavouras, S. A., ... Moreno, L. A. (2015). Total fluid intake of children and adolescents: Cross-sectional surveys in 13 countries worldwide. *European Journal of Nutrition*, 54 (2), 57–67. https://doi.org/10.1007/s00394-015-0946-6.

Jéquier, E., & Constant, F. (2010). Water as an essential nutrient: The physiological basis of hydration. *European Journal of Clinical Nutrition*, 64(2), 115–123. https://doi.org/10.1038/ejcn.2009.111.

Leatherman, T. L., & Goodman, A. (2005). Coca-colonization of diets in the Yucatan. *Social Science & Medicine*, 61(4), 833–846. https://doi.org/10.1016/j.socscimed.2004.08.047.

Lemus, J. (2019). *El agua o la vida: Otra guerra ha comenzado* [*Water or life: Another war has started*]. Editorial Grijalbo.

Lineamientos 2010 (Acuerdo mediante el cual se establecen los lineamientos generales para el expendio o distribución de alimentos y bebidas en los establecimientos de consumo escolar de los planteles de educación básica [General guidelines for the distribution or sales of food and drinks by retailers within basic education schools]) (2010). Diario Oficial de la Federación: Órgano del Gobierno Constitucional de los Estados Unidos Mexicanos.

Lineamientos 2014 (Acuerdo mediante el cual se establecen los lineamientos generales para el expendio y distribución de alimentos y bebidas preparados y procesados en las escuelas del Sistema Educativo Nacional [Guidelines for the sales and distribution of prepared and processed food and drinks in the Mexican national education system]) (2014). Diario Oficial de la Federación: Órgano del Gobierno Constitucional de los Estados Unidos Mexicanos.

Malik, V. S., Popkin, B. M., Bray, G. A., Després, J.-P., & Hu, F. B. (2010). Sugar-sweetened beverages, obesity, type 2 diabetes mellitus, and cardiovascular disease risk. *Circulation*, 121 (11), 1356–1364. https://doi.org/10.1161/CIRCULATIONAHA.109.876185.

Mazari-Hiriart, M., Espinosa, A. C., López-Vidal, Y., Arredondo-Hernández, R., Díaz-Torres, E., & Equihua-Zamora, C. (2010). Visión integral sobre el agua y la salud [A holistic approach to the relation between water and health]. In B. Jiménez-Cisneros, M. L. Torregrosa y Armentia, & L. Aboites-Aguilar (eds.), *El agua en México: Cauces y encauces* (pp. 291–315). Academia Mexicana de Ciencias.

Nagata, J. M., Barg, F. K., Valeggia, C. R., & Bream, K. D. W. (2011). Coca-colonization and hybridization of diets among the Tz'utujil Maya. *Ecology of Food and Nutrition*, 50 (4), 297–318. https://doi.org/10.1080/03670244.2011.568911.

Nash, J. (2007). Consuming interests: Water, rum, and Coca-Cola from ritual propitiation to corporate expropriation in highland Chiapas. *Cultural Anthropology*, 22(4), 621–639. https://doi.org/10.1525/can.2007.22.4.621.

Negoianu, D., & Goldfarb, S. (2008). Just add water. *Journal of the American Society of Nephrology*, 19(6), 1041–1043. https://doi.org/10.1681/ASN.2008030274.

Nestlé (2003). *Nestlé and water: Sustainability, protection, stewardship*. https://www.nestle.com/sites/default/files/asset-library/documents/reports/csv%20reports/water/sustainability_protection_stewardship_english.pdf.

Nestlé (2007). *The Nestlé water management report.* https://www.nestle.com/sites/defa ult/files/asset-library/documents/library/documents/environmental_sustainability/water-management-report-mar2007-en.pdf.

Opel, A. (1999). Constructing purity: Bottled water and the commodification of nature. *Journal of American Culture*, 22(4), 67–76.

Ortega-Avila, A. G., Papadaki, A., & Jago, R. (2018). Exploring perceptions of the Mexican Sugar-Sweetened Beverage Tax among adolescents in north-west Mexico: A qualitative study. *Public Health Nutrition*, 21(3), 618–626. https://doi.org/10.1017/S1368980017002695.

Ortega Castañeda, A. d. J. (2016). *Los factores determinantes del aumento del consumo de agua embotellada en México: Análisis desde el enfoque de políticas públicas* [*Factors influencing the rise in bottled water consumption in Mexico: A public policy analysis*]. Centro de Investigación y Docencia Económicas, A.C. Ciudad de México.

Pacheco-Vega, R. (2015). Agua embotellada en México: De la privatización del suministro a la mercantilización de los recursos hídricos [Bottled water in Mexico: Privatising supply and commodifying water]. *Espiral*, 22(63), 221–263.

Perrier, E. T., Armstrong, L. E., Bottin, J. H., Clark, W. F., Dolci, A., Guelinckx, I., ... Péronnet, F. (2020). Hydration for health hypothesis: A narrative review of supporting evidence. *European Journal of Nutrition*. https://doi.org/10.1007/s00394-020-02296-z.

Piernas, C., Barquera, S., & Popkin, B. M. (2014). Current patterns of water and beverage consumption among Mexican children and adolescents aged 1–18 years: Analysis of the Mexican National Health and Nutrition Survey 2012. *Public Health Nutrition*, 17(10), 2166–2175. https://doi.org/10.1017/S1368980014000998.

Popkin, B. M., D'Anci, K. E., & Rosenberg, I. H. (2010). Water, hydration, and health. *Nutrition reviews*, 68(8), 439–458. https://doi.org/10.1111/j.1753-4887.2010.00304.x.

Race, K. (2012). 'Frequent sipping': Bottled Water, the will to health and the subject of hydration. *Body & Society*, 18(3–4),72–98. https://doi.org/10.1177/1357034X12450592.

Rampersaud, G. C., Pereira, M. A., Girard, B. L., Adams, J., & Metzl, J. D. (2005). Breakfast habits, nutritional status, body weight, and academic performance in children and adolescents. *Journal of the American Dietetic Association*, 105(5), 743–760. https://doi.org/10.1016/j.jada.2005.02.007.

Reporte Indigo (2017). México compra más Coca Cola que cualquier otro país del mundo [Mexicans buy more Coca Cola that people in any other country around the globe]. *Reporte Indigo.* https://www.reporteindigo.com/reporte/mexico-compra-mas-coca-que-cualquier-otro-pais/.

Rivera, J. A., Muñoz-Hernández, O., Rosas-Peralta, M., Aguilar-Salinas, C. A., Popkin, B. M., & Willett, W. C. (2008). Consumo de bebidas para una vida saludable: Recomendaciones para la población [Beverage consumption for a healthy life: Recommendations for the Mexican population]. *Salud Pública de México*, 50(2), 173–195. https://doi.org/10.1590s0036-36342008000200011.

Russell, C., Baker, P., Grimes, C., Lindberg, R., & Lawrence, M. A. (2022). Global trends in added sugars and non-nutritive sweetener use in the packaged food supply: Drivers and implications for public health. *Public Health Nutrition*, 26(5), 952–964. https://doi.org/10.1017/S1368980022001598.

Sepúlveda, J., Valdespino, J. L., & García-García, L. (2006). Cholera in Mexico: The paradoxical benefits of the last pandemic. *International Journal of Infectious Diseases*, 10(1), 4–13. https://doi.org/10.1016/j.ijid.2005.05.005.

Shiva, V. (2016). *Water wars: Privatization, pollution, and profit.* North Atlantic Books.

Solís, A. (2017). Agua embotellada, el negocio multimillonario que México no necesita [Bottled water, the multimillion business that Mexico does not need]. *Forbes México.* https://www.forbes.com.mx/agua-embotellada-el-negocio-multimillonario-que-mexico-no-necesita/.

statista (2013). Annual per capita consumption of Coca-Cola's beverage products from 1991 to 2012, by country. https://www.statista.com/statistics/271156/per-capita-consumption-of-soft-drinks-of-the-coca-cola-company-by-country/.

statista (n.d.). Per capita consumption of carbonated soft drinks in 2019 in the ten most populated countries worldwide. https://www.statista.com/statistics/505794/cds-per-capita-consumption-in-worlds-top-ten-population-countries/#statisticContainer.

Stevano, S. (2014). *Women's work, food and household dynamics: A case study of Northern Mozambique* [PhD, SOAS University of London].

Stookey, J. D., Constant, F., Popkin, B. M., & Gardner, C. D. (2008). Drinking water is associated with weight loss in overweight dieting women independent of diet and activity. *Obesity*, 16(11), 2481–2488. https://doi.org/10.1038/oby.2008.409.

Stuckler, D., McKee, M., Ebrahim, S., & Basu, S. (2012). Manufacturing epidemics: The role of global producers in increased consumption of unhealthy commodities including processed foods, alcohol, and tobacco. *PLOS Medicine*, 9(6), e1001235. https://doi.org/10.1371/journal.pmed.1001235.

Swyngedouw, E. (2005). Dispossessing H_2O: The contested terrain of water privatization. *Capitalism Nature Socialism*, 16(1), 81–98. https://doi.org/10.1080/1045575052000335384.

Tortolero, A. (2000). *El agua y su historia: México y sus desafíos hacia el siglo XXI* [*Water and history: Mexico and its challenges towards the XXI century*]. Siglo XXI Editores.

Tourliere, M. (2015). El agua embotellada, el gran negocio del Siglo XXI [Bottled water, the business of the XXI century]. *Proceso.* https://www.proceso.com.mx/422619.

Valtin, H. (2002). "Drink at least eight glasses of water a day." Really? Is there scientific evidence for "8 × 8"? *American Journal of Physiology-Regulatory, Integrative and Comparative Physiology*, 283(5), R993–R1004. https://doi.org/10.1152/ajpregu.00365.2002.

Walsh, C. (2018). *Virtuous waters: Mineral springs, bathing, and infrastructure in Mexico.* University of California Press.

Wilder, M. (2010). Water governance in Mexico: Political and economic aperatures [sic] and a shifting state-citizen relationship. *Ecology and Society*, 15(2). http://www.jstor.org/stable/26268136.

7 Food Through Schools

What Futures?

Santa Rosa is located 40 kilometers northwest from Veracruz City, the largest city in the state of Veracruz, Mexico. The route follows 25 kilometers of highway and 15 kilometers of a backroad. I drove this route most of the days during my fieldwork. The 15-kilometer backroad was always interesting. At almost every speed bump, food in different forms was for sale. Near the first speed bump, fishermen sold recently caught *mojarras* [white fishes] from the river behind us. Meters ahead, small plastic bags with coconut flesh and peeled sugar canes, and industrial candies, snacks and sugary drinks were equally found displayed for sale aside the road.

Sugar cane fields dominate the landscape for the last 10 kilometers of the backroad to Santa Rosa. April and May are the final months of sugar cane harvesting. The *zafra*—as the sugar cane harvest season is known in Mexico—stirs the lives of people in Santa Rosa. Families are more affluent between November and May, which can be appreciated in the higher circulation and consumption of food products. During the zafra, roads equally bustle. The 15-kilometer backroad to Santa Rosa is usually completed in 15 minutes. Yet if trucks loaded with sugar cane are on the road, as happens commonly during the zafra, the travel time increases to nearly half an hour.

On my third visit to Emiliano Zapata Primary School in late April 2016, I drove behind a sugar cane-loaded truck. The slow driving *forced me* to pay attention to the labor performed by workers in the fields. Their faces were covered by a layer of sweat and ashes—in Mexico sugar cane is still burnt before cutting it. Making piles with the hand-cut canes laid on the ground and loading them onto trucks is rough labor; especially considering what workers are paid for it. Work in the school kitchen is, albeit different, equally tough. The cooks at Emiliano Zapata Primary School, for example, worked strenuously under difficult conditions for little money. The labor that goes into producing food and the conditions surrounding its production, however, are commonly obliterated in 'healthy eating' policy.

In the healthy lifestyles policies launched to 'fight' obesity in Mexico, food is reduced to a biological object. This book has offered a critique to this narrow view on food and its relation to health. It also showed how corporate interests have significantly shaped, and benefited from, the idea of healthy lifestyles and the framing of food it enables.[1] The analysis of policy documents and corporate

DOI: 10.4324/9781003356264-7

reports presented in Chapter 3 revealed the mechanisms through which market forces significantly shaped language in obesity policy. Chapters 4 and 6 showed how corporate interests are disseminated through the deployment of the discourses surrounding healthy lifestyles. These three chapters laid out the argument of this book. Together, Chapters 3, 4 and 6 demonstrated how 'healthy lifestyles' has aided in transferring the responsibility for obesity from its structural roots into the hands of individuals, and to expand market interests in the name of health.

As a tool of government, or what I have analytically framed in this book as a *dispositif*, healthy lifestyles depicts subjects as well-resourced, rational decision-making individuals who need to look after their own health. This ideal subject is one who invests time and resources and follows public health advice to insure themselves against the risks intrinsic to development and a modern life. This book situated this construction in the economic and political context from where it is commonly detached. In Mexico, as Chapters 1 and 2 showed, this type of subjectivity was enabled by market-driven policy change, the downsizing of the state and by new—market-influenced—forms of theorizing, researching and managing health. With a favorable policy environment, transnational food and drink corporations expanded their presence in Mexico, which became both an important market and a crucial provider of natural resources and labor.

In this context of structural change, the school was positioned as *the* ideal space to 'fight' obesity, mainly through the promotion of healthy eating and food regulations. Mainstream literature ascertained the pertinence of these strategies in obesity prevention, which informed policy development. This book has shown, adding to this literature, how—despite multiple difficulties—healthy eating policies have been partly successful in changing *some* consumption behaviors *within* schools. As Chapter 6 detailed, for instance, the consumption of *refrescos* in some schools decreased after the implementation of the *Lineamientos* in 2010. This policy, however, has not changed children's fondness for *refrescos*, particularly Coca-Cola, which are still widely consumed outside of school hours.[2] However, the book's goal was beyond exploring whether this policy works or does not work. My intention was to shed light on the complex dynamics surrounding policy implementation and to highlight the cultural and economic dimensions of food that are commonly overlooked, both in mainstream obesity literature and in the wider public debate.

Ethnography was central to the making of this book. Yet I would not claim it to be an ethnography. Reasons abound. Fieldwork length, my "closeness" to what I researched, my lack of "formal" training in anthropology and my own analysis could, for instance, be used as arguments against any claim of having produced an ethnography. I would then say that my ethnographic approach to the study of healthy lifestyles enabled me to "construct" data through day-to-day and localized interactions and practices around food. Through these data, and the "thick descriptions" (Geertz, 1973) written upon their analysis, this book has offered an alternative perspective on what 'healthy' eating policies *do* in schools, and how their normative character is resisted in the everyday food practices in these spaces. It also challenged the dominant narrative that blames teachers, students and families for their unwillingness to be 'healthy', 'responsible' citizens.

The time I spent observing food being produced, sold and consumed in schools, and the conversations I had with multiple actors involved in these processes—and in their regulation, afforded me a grasp of the complexity surrounding the implementation of healthy eating policy. Such complexity is perhaps not a surprise. Policy implementation is always a messy process. Yet what makes healthy eating policy particularly complex is the multiple roles food plays—as this book widely documented—in the lives of people, and in schools, in Mexico. These complex processes around food should also be considered in the making of healthy eating policy.[3]

My introductory fieldwork vignettes in Chapter 1 were thus intended to draw the readers' attention to the fact that food in Mexican schools is much more than "energy", as it has been conceptualized by policymakers. Instead, school food practices embody culture, labor, money and, foremost, politics. I further expanded on this point in Chapter 5 showing how the local economic and cultural conditions surrounding schools shape the ways in which teachers, students and cooks engage with and speak about food. My aim was, partly, to speak against the "ideal" construction of *the school*—note my emphasis on the singular—that prevails across policy and other discursive spaces where the solutions to obesity are proposed (Chapter 3).

The idea that schools are, at the same time, "factories of obese people" and thus the spaces to 'fight' obesity *par excellence*, needs to be reconsidered and critically debated (see also Gard, 2010; Gard & Pluim, 2014). One of the main arguments used to justify its construction as an "anti-obesity" site, is that the school is a "closed and controlled" space, as some of the policymakers I interviewed stated. Mexican schools are physically delimited by either fences or walls, depending on what a school can afford. Yet far from being "closed and controlled", they are porous spaces where discourses and material objects flow outwards and inwards. Schools are the point of encounter between the broader political project of the state and corporations, the beliefs and knowledges of the school staff and the private and intimate life of families.

Nothing exemplifies this better than teachers', parents', students' and cooks' practices around food. When a lunchbox or a plastic bag with home-made food is brought inside the school, a whole system of household ideas regarding food and cooking crosses the school's physical boundaries. Corporations penetrate the life of schools through material objects, like Nestlé's "Eatwell Plate", which display their logos and their perspectives on how to be a 'healthy' person. The state made its way into the community's, families' and students' lives through curriculum content, and policies like the *Lineamientos*. Mothers' and grannies' cooking knowledges enter schools to compete with the ideas about 'nutrition' and 'health' presented within the materials of national curriculum and health-promotion programs. This is why, following Appadurai (1981), I have proposed that in future policymaking schools need to be considered not as "obesogenic environments", but as gastro-political spaces where struggles over the meanings and economics of food are always at stake.

To elaborate my critique of the idea of schools as sites to change eating behavior in the name of 'fighting' obesity, I approached schools as historically, politically, geographically and culturally bounded spaces. Schools, as Chapter 2 showed, have played pivotal roles in the management of the Mexican population. For example, in post-revolutionary Mexico, schools aided—although with nuances and resistances—to build and enlarge the state and to transform a predominantly rural population into a trained workforce. Schools are not silos; they exist within a community and are entangled in larger power dynamics. There is not one single model of *the school*. Schools are diverse and, while they share commonalities (e.g., a national curriculum and a set of regulatory policies), each school is different.

The preparation, sale and consumption of food in schools consequently occurs in multiple ways. In Emiliano Zapata Primary School, Doña Martha, Moni, Beatriz and Angela worked relentlessly to feed students with nurturing, real food. The harsh conditions surrounding the school kitchen were overcame day-to-day by these four women through collective work and cooking knowledges. Ingredients were always scarce. Yet the cooks never let a hungry stomach go empty. The conditions surrounding the school (its location in a small rural community; the size of the school; abundant labor; a strong sense of community) enabled this way of engaging with food. The consumption of food in Benito Juárez Primary School was, naturally, framed under different logics. Nearly 1,000 students needed to be offered food in this school. The number of parents or grandparents delivering food to students during the break was considerably less here compared with Emiliano Zapata Primary School. Time and space were organized very differently. Hand-made foods were also prepared and offered on-site in this school, yet the profit-driven model under which food was provisioned required that ultra-processed products were also on sale. These products, as Chapter 5 narrated, are not only good for increasing profit margins but are also convenient from a labor perspective.

The *Lineamientos* establishes what food is to be produced in schools, how and by whom. Some positive, at times ephemeral, outcomes have been yielded by this policy (Chapter 6). Its "food-as-energy" and nutrient-centered focus has nevertheless also aided to stigmatize real food in schools. Like most healthy eating policies in schools, the *Lineamientos* silences the contextual meanings and divergent uses of food and promotes an individualistic view on food choices and health (see Trapp, 2022). Another problem with the food-as-energy discourse underpinning healthy eating policy is that it has enabled corporations to influence, as Chapter 3 showed, the making of policy. Drawing on this discourse, for instance, corporations were able to weaken the scope of the *Lineamientos*. As a policy that is focused on nutrients, the *Lineamientos* stigmatizes real food – such as *masa*-based foods – because they are "high in fats". Yet at the same time, this same framing enabled corporations to keep their ultra-processed products in schools by reducing the packaging size of their products.[4]

Through the "thick descriptions" of how *real* food comes to exist in schools offered in this book, I challenged this reductionist view on food and its relation to health—what Scrinis (2013) calls "nutritionism"—underpinning healthy eating policy. A change in how food is conceptualized in policy is therefore needed. Scrinis' (2013) proposal to transition from the current "nutritional reductionism" to a "food quality paradigm" is pertinent here. The latter, Scrinis (2013, pp. 215–216) suggests, defines foods primarily in terms of their nutrient composition, whereas the former considers "food production and processing quality, cultural-traditional knowledge, and sensual-practical experiences, as well as the nutritional-scientific analysis of nutrients, foods, and dietary patterns". The "food quality paradigm" brings back the social dimension of food that is obscured under the dominant "nutritional reductionist" paradigm. This book offered a critique of the former, but also intended to offer the reader a broader perspective of the multiple roles that food has in schools, and in the communities surrounding them. Hence my emphasis on labor and the economic significance of food.

Drawing upon his "food quality paradigm", Scrinis (2013) proposes an alternative to conventional food classification systems. Instead of focusing on nutrients and their biological functions, Scrinis suggests that classification should be made based on the "levels and intensity of processing" and "categories of ingredients" (pp. 218–219). Similarly, the NOVA classification, developed by a group of Brazilian nutrition epidemiologists led by Carlos A. Monteiro (Monteiro, 2009; Monteiro et al., 2010), also proposes a classification of foods based on their level and form of processing. The NOVA classification has become a critical tool for the analysis of the healthiness of foods and products, and has been used in the making of nutrition policy around the world (Mialon et al., 2018).

The adoption of this broader food classifications in the making of eating policy may contribute to more culturally-contextualize strategies. With a focus on the cultural, contextual process of *cooking*, rather than on abstract nutrients, for instance, this policy would be fairer for the multiplicity of realities in which food comes to exist in schools across Mexico. For example, the *empanadas, tostadas, gorditas* and *picaditas* that are widely consumed in schools across Veracruz would not be labelled as 'unhealthy' just because they are *masa*-made and contain some form of fat. Instead, the hard labor that goes into their making could be recognized and celebrated. Furthermore, this more-comprehensive food classification would facilitate the complete ban of ultra-processed products from schools. Why? Simply because they are not foods, but *industrial edible products* that have become widely consumed due to aggressive marketing and market-driven policies.[5]

I situated this research in a temporality I called "neoliberal Mexico". At the risk of annoying readers—neoliberal is widely and vaguely used in the social sciences (for critiques of this use, see Dean, 2014; Ferguson, 2010; Ong, 2007; Peck & Tickell, 2002; Springer, 2012)—I took this approach to emphasize that the production of both obesity and healthy lifestyles was enabled by the adoption of market-driven policies, the downsizing of the welfare state, a more in-depth integration with the United States and changes in the management and funding of scientific research that took place after the early 1980s. In Chapters 1 and 2, I described the emergence of this "neoliberal form of government" and its detrimental effects on the day-to-day lives and the health of the Mexican population.

The relation between the state and the population changed significantly with the adoption of the neoliberal form of government. This was evident in the conceptualization and operationalization of social policy. In a welfare economy, social policy is primarily redistributive. It seeks to counterweight the negative effects of economic processes through the provision of material resources (Foucault, 2008). Categorized as paternalistic and ineffective, this form of social policy is eroded under neoliberalism. Instead, "empowerment" emerged as the framework of social policy. Under this logic, the role of social policy is not to provide aid, but to encourage people to find the means and resources to satisfy their needs (Gupta, 2012; Sharma, 2008). The obesity and healthy eating policies discussed in this book are underpinned by this logic of empowerment: they tell people what they should do to be 'healthy', yet little is done to improve the material conditions under which food comes to exist.[6]

At the end of a focus groups interview I had with the Doñitas at Emiliano Zapata Primary School in late June 2016, I asked them if they wanted to ask or add anything else. With poise, Beatriz asked for "support [*apoyo*]", both for them and the schools. She did not specify what type of support, but I could be certain that Beatriz was claiming for financial support and for better working conditions. Beatriz made this claim, because she thought that I could voice her petition to be heard at a high "level". Precarity is the word that better describes the conditions under which food came to exist in the kitchen in this school. In previous chats while we were cooking together, the Doñitas used to emphasize the lack of a ceiling fan and kitchenware and the scarcity of cooking ingredients.

Benito Juárez Primary School was better equipped than Emiliano Zapata Primary School, which, to an extent, made the provisioning of food to children less complicated. Yet the "business-oriented" model under which the school canteen operated enabled the sale of unhealthful products and disadvantaged some students. More than once I observed, and heard of, children starving during the school day because they did not have money to buy food. They were lucky when other children shared their food, which occurred often. This, unfortunately, was not new to me. I witnessed hunger in schools many times during the five years I worked in education in Veracruz. In obesity and healthy eating policies, as I discussed in Chapter 5, it is implied that in schools, food is already *there*, available for children to consume. It is also assumed that all children have the means to buy food while in schools. But this is not always the case.

Since the mid-2000s, the provisioning of food in schools has become a popular research topic globally. Scholars from across disciplines (e.g., historians, nutrition scientists, sociologists, epidemiologists, educators) have investigated—both from mainstream and critical perspectives—how different countries feed children in schools (Berggren et al., 2021; Gaddis, 2020; Gaddis & Jeon, 2020; Illøkken et al., 2021; Levine, 2008; Moffat & Gendron, 2019; Pech, 2022; Poppendieck, 2010); the link between food education and school meal programs and obesity (Babashahi et al., 2021; Earl, 2018; Leahy et al., 2022; Nestle, 2013; Oostindjer et al., 2017) and the connections between school meals and food systems change (Cairns, 2018; Guitart et al., 2014; Merçon et al., 2018; Powell & Wittman, 2018). While diverse, this literature highlights that material resources and collective organization are needed to facilitate students the access to real food in schools. The school food–sustainability–health connection is another recurrent theme across part of this research, which has gained importance as research has demonstrated the impact our food consumption practices have on the environment and the effects of environmental change on human health.

Thus, better policies are needed to reduce the consumption of industrial edible products and to facilitate the consumption of real food in schools, which may eventually contribute to improving children's bodily health. Of course, it is easy, and perhaps meaningless, to make statements of this kind. But there is, I think, no harm in proposing ways to improve policy. In line with the argument of this book, putting in place a more culturally oriented school food policy could be considered a good starting point. Yet broader efforts to, for instance, improve working conditions of school cooks and to solve the harsh conditions that some Mexican schools face in terms of infrastructure, services and budget are also urgently needed.

As I described in Chapter 2, the production, sale and consumption of food in Mexican schools has been regulated since the 1930s. Throughout subsequent decades, several isolated attempts to provide food to children via schools have been part of broader food and nutrition policies, aimed primarily at alleviating poverty. However, a free, government-led school meal program has never existed in Mexico.[7] I am not suggesting that a school meal program is the panacea for obesity in Mexico. However, I do consider—from my professional, research and personal experiences with food in schools in Mexico—that a social policy of this type, in synergy with other structural policies aimed at improving the living conditions and health of the population, could help to improve access to healthful, handmade food to children in schools. Given the wildly complex politics in Mexico, the problem is how to frame and implement a policy of this type without it becoming just *one more* policy.

What I have proposed in this conclusion—the making of a more culturally-sensitive school food policy and the creation of a form of free, government-led school meal program—may not be entirely unattainable under the current political context and policy environment in Mexico. In 2018, Andrés Manuel López Obrador, a center-left politician who has been labelled as a "populist", was elected as president of Mexico. López Obrador's landslide win was perceived to be the result of his promise to tackle the social inequalities and corruption practices triggered by neoliberalism (Mattiace, 2019; Olvera, 2020). In line with this rhetoric—which has been widely criticized and deemed as a risk for Mexican democracy (Dresser, 2022; Reich, 2020; Sánchez-Talanquer & Greene, 2021)—the López Obrador government has increased spending in social programs, launched policies to re-positioning the state as a central actor in government and, in the public health space, backed policies that had not been supported by previous administrations because they threatened private interests.[8] It is beyond the scope of this book to evaluate current political rhetoric and government performance. The interested reader will find enough material to make their own mind. My intention is only to highlight that the current policy environment is favorable to advocate for more equitable actions to feed children in schools. In the end, I wrote this book to make Beatriz's voice heard.

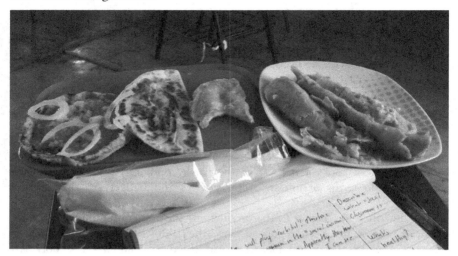

Figure 7.1 Plates with *antojitos* in a classroom at Emiliano Zapata Primary School. Photo by the author.

On my third visit to Emiliano Zapata Primary School on April 27, 2016, I arrived at Santa Rosa later than usual after slowly driving behind the cane-loaded truck. The main street in town was also busy. Children and their parents were happily running in a circuit in what seemed to be a race. I parked one block away from the school, walked towards the gate and joined some teachers who were seated on the sidewalk in front of the gate. It was a premium spot. The race, I was told, was part of the Children's Day celebrations: it was a day for fun and sharing.

By 10:00 am, after the race had finished, students entered their classrooms. It was time to share the homemade foods, and other products, they had brought in. Ángel, the fifth-grade teacher I was talking with, invited me to join his group. As we walked towards his classroom, Ángel said that that day he had been "relaxed" with the "regulations" because it was a special celebration. However, he stressed, on "normal days" he was "strict with the rules". Although I had already built rapport—mainly because the school community regarded me as an "insider"—I perceived that Ángel was trying to justify the abundance of *masa*-based foods, *refrescos* and candies in the classroom.

Almost immediately after I sat in one of the old classroom desks, a group of students approached me with a container full of *enchiladas*. One of them handed me a white ceramic plate and asked me how many *enchiladas* I wanted. I asked for three. Another group offered me sliced cucumbers and *jícamas* [Mexican yam bean] in small plastic bags. Generously, they wanted me to take one bag of each one. I took the *jícamas* only. Other students came to me with containers with *empanadas, picaditas* and *quesadillas*. They were looking for a spare plate to serve me one of each. The disposable plates were over. Resourcefully, a kid grabbed the lid of one of the containers, handed it to me and asked me to help myself.

The straightforwardness of this "improvised plate", and the food practices around it, kept me thinking for many years after I finished my fieldwork. In the end, I decided to interpret it as an alternative against the normativity of the project of governing through 'healthy lifestyles'. This modest, yet clever, improvised plate contrasts with the scrupulous, colorful design of Nestlé's "Eatwell Plate" (see Figure 1.1). The two plates represent two contrasting perspectives on food and its relation to health, and, crucially, two forms of social organization. Nestlé's "Eatwell Plate" was developed on scientific evidence provided by Nestlé's sponsored nutrition-related research and was endorsed by experts and by government and non-government entities as an optimal vehicle to 'educate' children to 'eat better'. This plate embodies the discourses that construct individuals as rational-and-well-resourced decision makers and food as an object to be quantified and regulated in the name of health.

The improvised plate, I think, embodies a sense of collectivism that, despite the lack of good government and the policies pushing them to act otherwise, Mexican people still have. The lid and the *antojitos* on it graciously exemplify that in Mexico *real* food, albeit complex, is a form of caring for the other.

Notes

1 To be clear, I have not proposed that corporations are using schools to advertise their products or to create more consumers. That view would be rather simplistic. The members of the school community, as I showed in Chapter 4, are actively resisting the corporate intentions to shape their lives. While it is undeniable that Nestlé's Eatwell Plate, for instance, is to some extent proof of how brands flow into schools in the name of promoting 'healthy lifestyles', I claimed that what is at stake is the silent dissemination of an "enterprise form" that, through a complex bio-political project, seeks to make rational and responsible individuals who can consume and still remain 'healthy'.

2 My teacher friends in southern Veracruz, with whom I worked for five years before starting my PhD, keep me informed of what is commonly sold in their schools. *Refrescos*, according to them, are still available in many schools in the region.

3 For an analysis of the ethical implications of "healthy eating efforts", see Barnhill & Bonotti (2021).

4 This point was explained to me by Ernesto, the director of the NGO Anti-Obesity Coalition. Clapp and Scrinis (2017, p. 579) have shown how corporations use "nutritional positioning and claims about the nutritional dimensions of their products" to "shape the regulatory environment in which they operate".

5 This conceptualization is influenced by my reading of Scrinis' (2013) discussion of the terminology used to classify food on the basis of processing quality. Otero and colleagues' discussion on the matter also shaped my decision to use the term "industrial edible products" (Otero et al., 2015).

6 Trying to change behavior through empowerment is not fundamentally bad, but it is dangerous, especially for the worse off whom, unlike the affluent, more often lack the time and economic resources to govern themselves. Sharma (2008, p. 27) offers a powerful critique of the empowerment "assemblage", showing how it became more pervasive as the World Bank deployed its 'development' initiatives throughout the Third World pursuing an "efficient and speedy market-centered growth".

7 Some of the food policies that have been put in place in Mexico from the early nineteenth century (see Fox, 1992; Ochoa, 2002) have targeted school-aged children.

However, a properly funded program aimed at equipping and enabling schools to feed children has never existed (also see Barquera et al., 2001)..

8   In the obesity space, as White and Barquera (2020) have discussed, the policy environment generated by the López Obrador government, which also has a majority in Congress, was one of the factors that favored the approval of a progressive food-warning-labels policy that had not gained the support of previous, "moderate conservative", governments.

References

Appadurai, A. (1981). Gastro-politics in Hindu South Asia. *American Ethnologist*, 8(3), 494–511. http://www.jstor.org/stable/644298.

Babashahi, M., Omidvar, N., Joulaei, H., Zargaraan, A., Zayeri, F., Veisi, E., Doustmohammadian, A., & Kelishadi, R. (2021). Scrutinize of healthy school canteen policy in Iran's primary schools: A mixed method study. *BMC Public Health* 21(1), 1566. https://doi.org/10.1186/s12889-021-11587-x.

Barnhill, A., & Bonotti, M. (2021). *Healthy eating policy and political philosophy: A public reason approach*. Oxford University Press.

Barquera, S., Rivera-Dommarco, J., & Gasca-Garcia, A. (2001). Políticas y programas de alimentación y nutrición en México [Food and nutrition policies and programs in Mexico]. *Salud Pública de México*, 43(5), 464–477. https://doi.org/10.1590/s0036-36342001000500011.

Berggren, L., Olsson, C., Rönnlund, M., & Waling, M. (2021). Between good intentions and practical constraints: Swedish teachers' perceptions of school lunch. *Cambridge Journal of Education*, 51(2), 247–261. https://doi.org/10.1080/0305764X.2020.1826406.

Cairns, K. (2018). Beyond magic carrots: Garden pedagogies and the rhetoric of effects. *Harvard Educational Review*, 88(4), 516–537.

Clapp, J., & Scrinis, G. (2017). Big Food, nutritionism, and corporate power. *Globalizations*, 14(4), 578–595. https://doi.org/10.1080/14747731.2016.1239806.

Dean, M. (2014). Rethinking neoliberalism. *Journal of Sociology*, 50(2), 150–163. https://doi.org/10.1177/1440783312442256.

Dresser, D. (2022). Mexico's dying democracy: AMLO and the toll of authoritarian populism. *Foreign Affairs*, 101(6), 74–90.

Earl, L. (2018). *Schools and food education in the 21st century*. Routledge.

Ferguson, J. (2010). The uses of neoliberalism. *Antipode*, 41(s1), 166–184. https://doi.org/10.1111/j.1467-8330.2009.00721.x.

Foucault, M. (2008). *The birth of biopolitics: Lectures at the Collège De France 1978–1979*, translated by G. Burchell. Picador

Fox, J. (1992). *The politics of food in Mexico: State power and social mobilization*. Cornell University Press.

Gaddis, J. E. (2020). *The labor of lunch: Why we need real food and real jobs in American public schools*. University of California Press.

Gaddis, J. E., & Jeon, J. (2020). Sustainability transitions in agri-food systems: insights from South Korea's universal free, eco-friendly school lunch program. *Agriculture and Human Values*, 37(4), 1055–1071. https://doi.org/10.1007/s10460-020-10137-2.

Gard, M. (2010). *The end of the obesity epidemic*. Routledge.

Gard, M., & Pluim, C. (2014). *Schools and public health. Past, present and future*. Lexington Books.

Geertz, C. (1973). *The interpretation of cultures*. Basic Books.

Guitart, D. A., Pickering, C. M., & Byrne, J. A. (2014). Color me healthy: Food diversity in school community gardens in two rapidly urbanising Australian cities. *Health & Place*, 26, 110–117. https://doi.org/10.1016/j.healthplace.2013.12.014.

Gupta, A. (2012). *Red tape: Bureaucracy, structural violence and poverty in India*. Duke University Press.

Illøkken, K. E., Johannessen, B., Barker, M. E., Hardy-Johnson, P., Øverby, N. C., & Vik, F. N. (2021). Free school meals as an opportunity to target social equality, healthy eating, and school functioning: experiences from students and teachers in Norway. *Food and Nutrition Research*, 65. https://doi.org/10.29219/fnr.v65.7702.

Leahy, D., Wright, J., Lindsay, J., Tanner, C., Maher, J., & Supski, S. (2022). School food in Australia—a dog's breakfast? In M. Gard, D. Powell, & J. Tenorio (eds.), *Routledge handbook of critical obesity studies* (pp. 166–176). Routledge.

Levine, S. (2008). *School lunch politics: The surprising history of America's favorite welfare program*. Princeton University Press.

Lineamientos 2010 (Acuerdo mediante el cual se establecen los lineamientos generales para el expendio o distribución de alimentos y bebidas en los establecimientos de consumo escolar de los planteles de educación básica [General guidelines for the distribution or sales of food and drinks by retailers within basic education schools]) (2010). Diario Oficial de la Federación: Órgano del Gobierno Constitucional de los Estados Unidos Mexicanos.

Lineamientos 2014 (Acuerdo mediante el cual se establecen los lineamientos generales para el expendio y distribución de alimentos y bebidas preparados y procesados en las escuelas del Sistema Educativo Nacional [Guidelines for the sales and distribution of prepared and processed food and drinks in the Mexican national education system]) (2014). Diario Oficial de la Federación: Órgano del Gobierno Constitucional de los Estados Unidos Mexicanos.

Mattiace, S. (2019). Mexico 2018: AMLO's hour. *Revista de Ciencia Política*, 39(2), 285.

Merçon, J., Morales, H., Nava Nasupcialy, K. N., & Ambrosio Montoya, M. (2018). La participación clave de las mujeres en huertos escolares de México. Reflexiones en torno a sus motivaciones, retos y aprendizajes. [Women's central role in school gardens in Mexico: Experiences, motivations, challenges and learnings]. In G. Zuluaga Sánchez, G. Catacora-Vargas, & E. Siliprandi (eds.), *Agroecología en femenino: Reflexiones from our experiences [Agroecology among women: Reflections from our experiences]* (pp. 159–180). SOCLA/CLACSO.

Moffat, T., & Gendron, D. (2019). Cooking up the "gastro-citizen" through school meal programs in France and Japan. *Food, Culture & Society*, 22(1), 63–77. https://doi.org/10.1080/15528014.2018.1547587.

Mialon, M., Sêrodio, P., & Scagliusi, F. B. (2018). Criticism of the NOVA classification: Who are the protagonists? *World Nutrition*, 9(3), 176–240. https://doi.org/10.26596/wn.201893176-240.

Monteiro, C. A. (2009). Nutrition and health. The issue is not food, nor nutrients, so much as processing. *Public Health Nutrition*, 12(5), 729–731. https://doi.org/10.1017/S1368980009005291.

Monteiro, C. A., Levy, R. B., Claro, R. M., Ribeiro de Castro, I. R., & Cannon, G. (2010). A new classification of foods based on the extent and purpose of their processing. *Cadernos de Saúde Pública*, 26(11), 2039–2049.

Nestle, M. (2013). School meals: A starting point for countering childhood obesity. *JAMA Pediatrics*, 167(6), 584–585. https://doi.org/10.1001/jamapediatrics.2013.404.

Ochoa, E. (2002). *Feeding Mexico: The political use of food since 1910*. Scholarly Resources Inc.

Olvera, A. J. (2020). México 2018: elección plebiscitaria, crisis neoliberal y proyecto populista [Mexico 2018: Plebiscite election, neoliberal crisis and populist project]. In G. Caetano & F. Mayorga (eds.), *Giros políticos y desafíos democráticos en América Latina: Enfoques de casos nacionales y perspectivas de análisis* [*Political turns and democratic challenges in Latin America: Approaches of national cases and analysis perspectives*] (pp. 115–142). CLACSO.

Ong, A. (2007). Neoliberalism as a mobile technology. *Transactions of the Institute of British Geographers*, 32(1), 3–8. https://doi.org/10.1111/j.1475-5661.2007.00234.x.

Oostindjer, M., Aschemann-Witzel, J., Wang, Q., Skuland, S. E., Egelandsdal, B., Amdam, G. V., Schjøll, A., Pachucki, M. C., Rozin, P., Stein, J., Lengard Almli, V., & Van Kleef, E. (2017). Are school meals a viable and sustainable tool to improve the healthiness and sustainability of children's diet and food consumption? A cross-national comparative perspective. *Critical Reviews in Food Science and Nutrition*, 57(18), 3942–3958. https://doi.org/10.1080/10408398.2016.1197180.

Otero, G., Pechlaner, G., Liberman, G., & Gürcan, E. (2015). The neoliberal diet and inequality in the United States. *Social Science & Medicine*, 142, 47–55. https://doi.org/10.1016/j.socscimed.2015.08.005.

Pech, A. (2022). *Au-delà de la cantine et du potager: ressources et freins à une éducation alimentaire des adolescent. es au collège. Étude du foodscape de trois collèges (France, Mexique)* [*Beyond the canteen and the vegetable garden: Enablers and barriers to food education for adolescents in secondary school. Study of the foodscape in three colleges (France, Mexico)*] [PhD, École normale supérieure de Lyon].

Peck, J., & Tickell, A. (2002). Neoliberalizing space. *Antipode*, 34(3), 380–404. https://doi.org/10.1111/1467-8330.00247.

Poppendieck, J. (2010). *Free for all: Fixing school food in America*. University of California Press.

Powell, L. J., & Wittman, H. (2018). Farm to school in British Columbia: Mobilizing food literacy for food sovereignty. *Agriculture and Human Values*, 35(1), 193–206. https://doi.org/10.1007/s10460-017-9815-7.

Reich, M. R. (2020). Restructuring health reform, Mexican style. *Health Systems & Reform*, 6(1), e1763114. https://doi.org/10.1080/23288604.2020.1763114.

Sánchez-Talanquer, M., & Greene, K. F. (2021). Is Mexico falling into the authoritarian trap? *Journal of Democracy*, 32(4), 56–71. https://doi.org/10.1353/jod.2021.005c.

Scrinis, G. (2013). *Nutritionism: The science and politics of dietary advice*. Columbia University Press.

Sharma, A. (2008). *Logics of empowerment: Development, gender, and governance in neoliberal India*. University of Minnesota Press.

Springer, S. (2012). Neoliberalism as discourse: Between Foucauldian political economy and Marxian poststructuralism. *Critical Discourse Studies*, 9(2), 133–147. https://doi.org/10.1080/17405904.2012.656375.

Trapp, M. M. (2022). Performing vegetable nutrition: Rethinking school food and health. *Culture, Agriculture, Food and Environment*, 44(2), 120–131. https://doi.org/10.1111/cuag.12297.

White, M., & Barquera, S. (2020). Mexico adopts food warning labels, why now? *Health Systems & Reform*, 6(1), e1752063. https://doi.org/10.1080/23288604.2020.1752063.

Index

Note: Page locators in *italics* refer to figures and "n" refers to notes.

public health 5, 33; critical 7; in Mexico
and U.S. influence 43–45; schools and
69, 155
public–corporate partnerships *see*
public–private partnerships
public–private partnerships 4, 20, 65–66,
80, 89–90, 94; *see also* corporate
bio-political project

Queremos Mexicanos Activos 66, 67,
75n10
quesadillas (food) xiv, 3, 14, 106–108,
114, 160,
quesillo (food) xiv, 3, 113

recipes 86–88
refrescos (drink) xiv, 7, 47, 127–130,
134–137; and obesity 135; *see also Coca*
refrigerio 132, 141–143
Reglamento 1934 45–46
Reglamento 1937 45–46
Reglamento 1962 46
Reglamento 1982 46–47, 68–69,
75n15, 105
revolving door 23n18
Rockefeller Foundation 43, 96
Rockwell, Elsie 121n5
Rose, Nikolas 83, 95

Sabritas 18, 106
Salinas, Carlos 8, 9, 38–39, 145; *see also*
form of government: neoliberal
saludable see healthy
sana/sano see healthy
sandwiches xi, 107, 127, 132, 140, 147n1
schools: as anti-obesity sites 34, 59, 69, 71,
119, 154–155; as gastro-political spaces
155; as historical and political spaces 20,
69, 102, 139, 155–156; and public
health interventions 22n15, 41; precarity
in 158; and government projects 40; and
modernization 41–42
school canteen xi, xii, 158; *see also cooperativa
escolar*
school food xi, 18, 45, 63, 108, 121n4,
159; and child health 22n15; and
families' economies 10, 105–106, 111;
as income 15, 46, 48, 68, 105–106,
115; and labor (*see* cooking: as labor),
management 102–103, 105; practices
16, 34, 81, 94, 155
school food policies in Mexico 6,
45–48, 67, 101; critique of 73,
116, 159

school infrastructure 33, 59, 71, 102–104,
159; lack of for feeding student
110–111; personal connections and
improvement of 120; and tap water
consumption 130 (see also water
fountains in schools)
school meal programs xi, 107; 158–159
Scrinis, Gyorgy 6, 22n14, 115, 156–157,
161n5
SEP (Secretaría de Educación Pública) xv, 41
SEV (Secretaría de Educación de Veracruz)
xv, 6, 13, 80, 129
shared responsibility 59, 65; discourse in
action 80–81
Sharma, Aradhana 161n6
SNTE (Sindicato Nacional de Trabajadores
de la Educación) 70; *see also* unions
Soberón, Guillermo 44; *see also*
FUNSALUD
social policy 8, 35, 39, 74, 159; neoliberalism
and 157–158
Sonrics 18
Spalding, Rose J. 38
state: corporatist 19, 34, 38; neoliberal 34,
19, 94–95; welfare 17, 58, 157
Stevano, Sara 47n8
sugar: consumption 62, 82, 88, 115, 140,
142, 127; decline in production and
migration 23n20; and free trade 11–12
sugar cane: as food 153; industry and local
economy 10, 11, 110, 112; production
of, in Mexico 10, 110, 153
sugar tax 23n23, 60, 73, 129–130, 134,
136, 139, 147n4
sugary drinks *see* carbonated-sugary drinks;
refrescos
SUMA 80, 96n1
SUMA-Nutrir 6, 20, 80–81, 101–102, 128,
143; *see also* public–private partnerships;
Nestlé: healthy lifestyles programs

tamales (food) 82, 144
teachers 2, 3, 4, 6, 7, 11, 13, 15, 41,
75n16, 92–93, 101, 104–105, 110–112,
137, 145; and food preparation
111–112; food sale 45–46, 105; as
political actors 33, 36, 40, 111, 120,
122n24; promoting dietary change and
modernity 42; role in promoting healthy
lifestyles 68–70, 80, 87, 89, 128, 130,
132, 140, 160; views on food options in
schools 106, 107–108, 113, 141–142
technocrats: political 38–39, 50n8; health
40, 49, 146

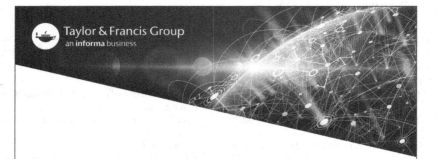